Aids to Operative Surgery

Graeme J. Poston

FRCS FRCSEd

Registrar, Department of Surgery,
Royal Postgraduate Medical School,
Hammersmith Hospital, London, UK

CHURCHILL LIVINGSTONE

EDINBURGH LONDON MELBOURNE AND NEW YORK 1987

CHURCHILL LIVINGSTONE
Medical Division of Longman Group UK Limited

Distributed in the United States of America by
Churchill Livingstone Inc., 1560 Broadway, New
York, N.Y. 10036, and by associated companies,
branches and representatives throughout the
world.

First published 1987
    Reprinted 1989
    Reprinted 1991

ISBN 0 443 03566 0

British Library Cataloguing in Publication Data
Poston, Graeme J.
    Aids to operative surgery.
    1. Surgery
    I. Title
    617   RD31

Library of Congress Cataloging in Publication Data
Poston, Graeme J.
    Aids to operative surgery.

    Includes bibliographies and index.
    1. Surgery, Operative — Handbooks, manuals, etc.
I. Title. [DNLM: 1. Surgery, Operative — handbooks.
WO 39 P858a]
RD32.P59   1986   617'.91   86-8320

Produced by Longman Singapore Publishers (Pte) Ltd
Printed in Singapore

Preface

This is not a textbook of operative surgery. Its aim is to aid in revising operative surgery to the level required for the Final FRCS examination in the United Kingdom, concentrating on those operations which are commonly asked about and general principles relating to more specialised procedures and operative problems. However, it should not be regarded as the definitive syllabus of operative surgery for the FRCS.

The anatomist Frank Stansfield described revising as 'learning' something for the first time the week before the examination', and the key to exam success as 'constant repetition'. I hope that by adopting the latter in describing operations, it is possible to avoid the former. The layout of the book is topographical: general, vascular, head and neck, cardiothoracic, upper gastrointestinal, hepatobiliary, colorectal, urological, orthopaedic and trauma surgery. Each description follows the same style to reinforce exam technique.

London, 1987   G.J.P.

Acknowledgements

I claim no originality for this text; most of these operations are long established in the surgical repertoire. This book is a distillate of the views of others, in particular the surgeons for whom I have worked.

I am especially grateful to the following members of staff of the Department of Surgery at the Royal Postgraduate Medical School for reading and constructively criticising the text: Professor L. H. Blumgart, Professor H. H. Bentall, Mr J. Spencer, Miss A. O. Mansfield, Mr J. A. Lynn, Mr C. B. Wood, Mr G. Williams and Mr R. C. Coombs. I would also like to thank my publishers, Churchill Livingstone, for their help and guidance with the preparation of this book.

I wish to thank Mrs Iris Fisher for the many hours spent in typing the manuscript and, finally, my wife June, for her unending patience in the many months of preparation. This book is dedicated to her.

Contents

Introduction

HOW TO USE THE BOOK

The layout of operations is constant throughout the book, and by following it, it will be possible for the reader to describe any operation from the removal of a sebaceous cyst to a major hepatic resection. There are often many ways of performing an operation, all of which are acceptable, but in order to keep within the brief of the 'Aids' series, I have described only one way of performing each procedure. However, if you wish to describe another way of doing an operation then write it down using the 'skeleton' described below. There may be other operations you wish to include in your revision and I suggest that you adopt a similar pattern for these.

HOW TO ANSWER QUESTIONS IN OPERATIVE SURGERY

An operation commences with preoperative preparation and the description should continue sequentially with specific points about anaesthesia, incision, approach, procedure and difficulties encountered, closure, postoperative management and postoperative complications. Questions may be phrased in a vague manner and the examiner may be trying to set a trap for the candidate; one of this type is to be asked to describe an operation like meniscectomy. The candidate commences at the incision describing the operation beautifully and logically, only to be failed at the end for forgetting to say that he would examine the patient preoperatively and mark the side. On the other hand, candidates may be reluctant to exasperate a tired examiner at the end of a long day by commencing on a long, drawn out description; usually examiners will interject in such cases and point out where they want the description to commence. If you adopt a step by step answer it becomes difficult to fall into any pitfalls of procedure.

PREOPERATIVE PREPARATION

Examine the patient and obtain informed consent, explaining any unusual outcomes such as colostomy or complications such as facial nerve palsy in parotidectomy. Mark the site and if the operation is ever on a structure which is bilateral, *mark the side.*

Special investigations
Those investigations which are necessary for safe anaesthesia (including sickle testing) and those specific to the disease concerned or operation should be described, including the amount of blood to be cross-matched.

Special preparation
Describe all procedures necessary to improve the technique or safety of the operation such as bowel preparation in colorectal surgery.

Antibiotic prophylaxis and steroid cover
Is it warranted and if so which drug or combination of antibiotics are indicated for this type of surgery?

Deep vein thrombosis
Does this procedure carry an increased risk of DVT (such as pelvic surgery) or are there any of the risk factors associated with DVT (smoking, oral contraceptives, age, etc.)?

Tubes
Should the patient be catheterised, have a drip or a nasogastric tube passed for this operation?

PRE-INCISION

Anaesthesia
Specify the type of anaesthesia employed, noting relevant points regarding agents and endotracheal intubation.

Position
Describe the positioning of the patient on the table and type of table (X-ray, Lloyd Davis supports, etc.) which you would use.

Skin preparation
Specify the extent, type of antiseptics used and placing of towels.

Position of surgeon
Describe the positioning of the surgeon, his assistants and where you would expect the scrub nurse to stand, reinforcing the impression that you have actually taken part in this procedure.

Incision
Specify the incision to be employed and acceptable alternatives. Justify your choice.

THE PROCEDURE

The approach
Describe the approach, noting anatomical landmarks and use of tissue planes (the examiner may wish you to avoid this and will usually indicate if so).

The procedure
Assess the pathology and any associated problems, especially expected coexistent pathology. Describe how *you* would do the operation, which sutures *you* would use, which instruments *you* would use.

Recognised problems
Note any common problems with this procedure and the techniques which are employed to deal with them.

Closure
Always describe methods of haemostasis and discuss whether or not drains are necessary. Remember the swab and instrument check and describe the closure *you* would use.

POSTOPERATIVE MANAGEMENT

Timing
Specify timing of removal of sutures, drains, tubes and dressings.

Specific instructions
Give specific instructions on postoperative management and care to be given to junior medical staff and nursing staff.

Special investigations
Describe special investigations relevant to the procedure (e.g. haemoglobin and transfusion, histology, microbiology, radiology and biochemistry).

Recognised complications
Describe recognised complications specific to the procedure, early and late and general complications of major surgery (DVT and PE, chest infection, wound infection, abscess, septicaemia, acute retention of urine, ileus etc.).

General surgery

PRINCIPLES OF PREVENTION OF SURGICAL SEPSIS
1. The problem
   (i) Wound infection
   (ii) Peritoneal infection
      a. Peritonitis
      b. Abscess
   (iii) Pulmonary infection
   (iv) Prosthesis infection
   (v) Septicaemia
   (vi) Pseudomembranous colitis
2. Sources
   (i) Autogenous ⎱ needs an innoculum of >10⁵
   (ii) Exogenous ⎰ bacteria
3. Factors
   (i) Virulence of organism and numbers/concentration of innoculum
   (ii) Local
      a. Surgical technique
      b. Drainage
      c. Ischaemia
      d. Obesity
      e. Foreign material
      f. Gut surgery
   (iii) General
      a. Age
      b. Immune status
      c. Pathology, especially malignancy
      d. Steroids
      e. Diabetes
      f. Cytotoxic chemotherapy
      g. Jaundice
      h. Uraemia
   (iv) Organism
      a. Aerobes ⎱ virulence and
      b. Anaerobes ⎰ pathogenicity

Methods of prevention
1. Prevent innoculation
    (i) Aseptic technique
    (ii) Theatre
        a. Minimise movements of personnel
        b. Air change with filter, laminar flow and positive
           pressure
    (iii) Surgical technique, care of tissues, haemostasis, no
          spillage, antiseptics
    (iv) Plastic drapes do not reduce wound infection
    (v) Bowel preparation (see colorectal surgery, page 116)
2. Antiseptics
    (i) Alcohol (70% Isopropyl)
        a. Bactericidal but evaporates and is short acting
        b. Avoid in wounds since neurotoxic
    (ii) Dyes
         Proflavine, gentian violet — useful with gram positive
         cocci except *Staphylococccus* and no use in slough
    (iii) Formaldehyde (noxytyalin)
          Releases 1% formaldehyde and is useful in peritoneal
          lavage
    (iv) Halogens
        a. Hypochlorite (Eusol, Miltons solution)
        b. Iodoforms (iodine in alcohol)
        c. Both bactericidal and sporicidal, including
           Staphylococcus. Limited by patient hypersensitivity
    (v) Phenols
        a. Hexochloraphane — of historic interest since
           introduced by Lister
        b. Problems: absorption may lead to neurotoxicity
        c. Staphylococcal resistance
    (vi) Quaternary ammonium (cetrimide, chlorhexidine)
        a. Bactericidal, not sporicidal
        b. Pseudomonas can grow in it!
    (vii) Silver sulphadiazine (flamazine)
          Will kill pseudonomas and useful in burns
3. Antibiotics
    (i) Prophylactic uses
        a. Appendicectomy
        b. Colorectal surgery
        c. Upper gut and hepatobiliary surgery
        d. Orthopaedic prosthesis surgery
        e. Risk of endocarditis following rheumatic fever
        f. Arterial surgery

  (ii) Disadvantages
    a. No compensation for poor surgery
    b. Masks signs of abscess
    c. Development of resistance; selection and emergence, drug tolerance and plasmid transmission
    d. Toxicity — specific organs, allergy and anaphylaxis, agranulocytosis, pyoderma gangrenosum, pseudomembranous colitis with overgrowth of *Clostridium difficile*
  (iii) When using an antibiotic always consider
    a. Is drainage better?
    b. Is lavage better?
    c. Is physiotherapy better?
  (iv) Always culture organisms and obtain sensitivity
  (v) Choice of antibiotic depends on
    a. Suspected organism
    b. Route of administration
    c. Route of metabolism/excretion
    d. Patient tolerance
  (vi) Antibiotic prophylaxis
    Use for the shortest possible time, therefore usually only two or three doses commencing with premedication or anaesthetic induction for up to 24 hours post surgery (if the course lasts longer than this then it should be considered a therapeutic procedure)
  (vii) Specific cases
    a. Upper gut surgery — Emergency surgery (see oversew of a perforated duodenal ulcer, page 94) Malignancy (see gastectomy, page 95) Obstruction (see laparotomy, page 100) Strangulation Opening the bowel electively
    b. Hepatobiliary (see cholecystectomy, page 102) — > 70 years old Within 4 weeks of biliary infection Jaundice Malignancy Bile duct surgery
    c. Appendicectomy (see page 117)

d. Small bowel — Obstruction (see laparotomy, page 100) Strangulation Crohn's disease

e. All colorectal surgery (see page 116)

f. Vascular surgery — Reconstruction using artificial materials (see principles of elective vascular reconstruction, page 28) Amputation for ischaemia (see below and above knee amputations, pages 40–43)

g. Cardiac surgery — Open heart surgery, especially with valve prostheses (see principles of cardiac surgery, page 74)

h. Thoracic surgery — Lung resection (see pneumonectomy, page 72)

i. Orthopaedic surgery for joint replacement (either systemic, topical irrigation or within cement) (see total hip replacement, page 174)

PRINCIPLES OF PREVENTION OF DEEP VEIN THROMBOSIS (DVT)

DVT

1. Incidence (including subclinical cases) by labelled fibrinogen studies
   (i) Major surgery, 40%
   (ii) Cerebovascular accident/multiple injuries, 60%
2. Aetiology
   Virchow's triad
   a. Blood — Increased viscosity
   Increased packed cell volume
   b. Flow — Stasis
   c. Vessel wall — Compression (operating table)
   Trauma
3. Risk groups
   (i) Female
   (ii) > 40 years old
   (iii) Smokers

(iv) Obese
(v) Oral contraceptive pill
(vi) Long general anaesthetic
(vii) Type of surgery
   a. Pelvic surgery
   b. Hip surgery
(viii) Malignant disease
(ix) Major long bone fracture and pelvic fracture
(x) Pelvic sepsis

Prophylaxis of DVT
1. Mechanical
  (i) Compression stocking
  (ii) Pulsion pneumatic compression
  (iii) Electrical calf muscle stimulation
  (iv) Foot pedals
  (v) Ankle rests to elevate calves
2. Pharmacological
  (i) "Mini dose" heparin, 5000 units subcutaneously twice daily from premedication to full mobilisation. Reduces the incidence of DVT from 40 to 10%.
  (ii) Dextran 70; peroperative infusion for up to 2 days postoperation. Reduces platelet adhesiveness and the incidence of DVT from 40 to 20%
    (Direct clinical comparison of Heparin and Dextran 70 shows Heparin to be significantly better)
  (iii) Aspirin, not proven to reduce DVT
  (iv) Problems
    a. All increase operative "ooze" of blood
    b. Dextran interferes with blood cross-matching and can impair renal function
3. Postoperative care
  (i) Early mobilisation
  (ii) Avoid calf compression and leg crossing
  (iii) Improve hydration
  (iv) Graduated compression stockings

Diagnosis of DVT
1. Clinical
  (i) Positive Homan's sign unreliable
  (ii) Swollen painful calf and leg
  (iii) Pulmonary embolism
2. Investigations
  (i) Doppler calf studies
  (ii) Plethysmography
  (iii) Venography
  (iv) Isotope labelled fibrinogen/streptokinase

Treatment of DVT
1. Anticoagulate
   Fully heparinise immediately and continue for 10 days,
   checking thrombin time and fully warfarinise for 6 months,
   checking prothrombin time regularly
2. Streptokinase
   Only if very large with imminent danger of embolism and
   not postoperatively or with a history of peptic ulceration
3. Thrombectomy
   If venogram suggests that it is not fixed
4. IVC plication or filter
5. Ancrod
   Experimental

Pulmonary embolism
1. Associated with ileofemoral and pelvic DVTs, although only
   30% have clinically proven DVTs
2. Accounts for 5% of hospital deaths
3. Usually occur 7–12 days post surgery
4. Effects
   (i) Minor
       a. Pleuritic chest pain
       b. Haemoptysis
       c. Pleural effusion ⎫ on chest X-ray
       d. Atelectasis ⎭
   (ii) Major
       a. Cardiopulmonary collapse
       b. Increased JVP
       c. Decreased cardiac output
       d. ECG changes — Lead 1-S wave
                          Lead 3-Q wave
                          T wave inversion
       e. Chest leads — Right side strain
5. Investigations
   (i) Chest X-ray
   (ii) ECG
   (iii) Baseline clotting screen prior to anticoagulation
   (iv) Ventilation perfusion isotope lung scan
   (v) Pulmonary angiography
   (vi) Increased LDH
6. Treatment
   (i) Medical
       a. Anticoagulate as for DVT
       b. Streptokinase
       c. Ancrod
   (ii) Surgery
       a. Caval interruption; plication/filter
       b. Trendelenberg pulmonary embolectomy

PRINCIPLES OF PREVENTION AND TREATMENT OF PULMONARY PROBLEMS DURING OPERATIONS

1. Patients at risk
   (i) Smokers
   (ii) Obese
   (iii) Elderly
   (iv) Chronic obstructive airways disease
   (v) Acute infection of respiratory tract
   (vi) Other pulmonary pathology (asthma, TB, carcinoma of bronchus)
2. Factors in airway narrowing
   (i) Reversible
      a. Secretion
      b. Wall thickening (partially reversible)
   (ii) Irreversible
      Airway collapse with loss of elasticity
3. Principles of preoperative management
   (i) Aims
      a. Identify risk and assess factors
      b. Minimise or eliminate effects of risk factors before, during and after surgery
   (ii) Method
      a. History and examination
      b. Chest radiology
      c. Lung function tests
      d. Blood gases
   (iii) Treatment
      a. Bronchodilators
      b. Systemic steroids
      c. Inhalation (steam, bronchodilators, steroids)
      d. Physiotherapy
      e. (Antibiotics)

Specific respiratory problems
1. Arterial hypoxaemia
   (i) Especially elderly with postoperative confusion
   (ii) Ventilation perfusion inadequacy with shunting
2. Atelectasis
   (i) Especially elderly and obese
   (ii) Reduces tidal volume
   (iii) Treat with physiotherapy
3. Gastric aspiration
   (i) Emergency surgery, especially for bowel obstruction (see laparotomy, page 100)
   (ii) Haematemesis
   (iii) Treat with steroids, antibiotics, physiotherapy and ventilation support

4. Pulmonary embolism (see page 9)
   (i) Risk groups (see page 7)
   (ii) Treat with anticoagulation
   (iii) In severe cases
     a. Streptokinase
     b. Trendelenberg pulmonary embolectomy
     c. IVC plication/filter
5. Pleural effusion
   (i) Occurs in 60% of upper abdominal operations (often subclinically)
   (ii) Increased risk
     a. Hypoalbuminaemia
     b. Subphrenic collections
     c. Embarrasses ventilation
6. Acute infection
   (i) Acute exacerbation of bronchitis
   (ii) Bacterial pneumonia
   (iii) Lung abscess
   (iv) Empyema (see drainage of empyema, page 73)

PRINCIPLES OF SKIN GRAFTING

Skin grafts may either be
   (i) Free
   (ii) Skin flaps
   (iii) Pedicled
   (iv) Free with microsurgical anastomosis
1. Free partial thickness (Thiersch)
   (i) Use on
     a. Large denuded areas
     b. Granulating wounds
     c. Site where contracture of the graft is of little cosmetic or functional consequence
   (ii) Advantage
     Takes easily
   (iii) Disadvantage
     Contractures which are inversely proportional to the thickness of the graft
2. Free full thickness (Wolfe)
   (i) Needs
     a. Strict asepsis
     b. Vascular recipient site
   (ii) Advantage
     No contracture, therefore better cosmesis
   (iii) Disadvantage
     a. No tolerance of sepsis
     b. Closure of donor site
   (iv) No free graft will take on tendon, bone, joint surface or within a mucosal cavity

3. Factors in graft survival
    (i) Skin applied to healthy granulating surface
    (ii) No subcutaneous fat transplanted
    (iii) Accurate apposition to granulating surface
    (iv) Immobilisation of graft
    (v) Revascularisation within 48 hours by capillary loops from granulation tissue
    (vi) Absence of infection (especially haemolytic *Streptococcus*)
    (vii) General health of patient
4. Graft failure due to
    (i) Failure of revascularisation
    (ii) Haematoma/seroma
    (iii) Poor immobilisation
    (iv) Infection
    (v) Poor recipient bed (bone, cartilage, tendon etc)
5. Technique of grafting
    (i) Partial thickness using dermatome (free hand, power, drum)
    (ii) Full thickness matching donor and recipient site and using scalpel to dissect out donor site
6. Skin flaps
    (i) Indications
        a. Poor recipient site
        b. Good cosmesis necessary
    (ii) Specific sites
        a. Eye lid
        b. Cheek
        c. Intra cavity
        d. Breast reconstruction
    (iii) Types
        a. Cutaneous pattern flap
        b. Axial
        c. Musculocutaneous
        d. Free with microsurgical anastomosis
        e. Pedicled flap
    (iv) Disadvantages of pedicled flaps
        a. May take several operations and months to move a flap from donor to recipient site
        b. Whereas free grafting performed at single operation
        c. May not match skin colour and hair
7. Free grafting with microsurgical anastomosis of vessels
    (i) Types of graft
        a. Cutaneous
        b. Myocutaneous
        c. Myo-osseocutaneous
        d. Osseocutaneous
    (ii) Specific donor sites

Type	Vascular basis
Ileo femoral	Superficial circumflex iliac vessels
Radial forearm	Radial artery
Deltopectoral	Anterior division of internal mammary vessels
Scalp	Superficial temporal vessels
Thoracodorsal	Lateral thoracic vessels
Foot	Dorsalis pedis and long saphenous vein
Greater omentum	Gastroepiploic vessels
(for surface cover	
or filling cavity)	

(iii) Technique
   a. Needs two patent veins for every artery of anastomosis
   b. Very accurate apposition with no tension and interrupted sutures with 9/0 prolene
   c. Very gentle tissue handling and meticulous dissection using jewellers instruments
   d. Full heparinisation of all vessels
   e. Nerve anastomoses — Excise all neuromata and use perineural sutures (see principles of management of nerve and tendon injury, page 199)
   f. Use operating microscope unless the vessels are > 2–3 mm in size, then use an operating loupe (× 2–4 magnification)
   g. Problems — Donor tissue is anaesthetic
               Graft failure due to:
               Poor vascularity
               Sutures under tension
               Vessel kinking
               Extrinsic pressure on vessels
               Haematoma
               Infection
   If failure is suspected then inject flourescein intravenously and observe the graft under ultraviolet light for evidence of fluorescence suggesting vascular viability

INGUINAL HERNIA REPAIR

1. In children
   (i) More common in boys
   (ii) Always indirect

(iii) Principles
  a. Often bilateral (incidence of right:left is 2:1)
  b. Often associated with abnormalities of descent
     (undescended and ectopic testis, see page 159)
  c. Often contains the ovary in girls under 2 years old
  d. High incidence of strangulation in the first few
     months of life
  e. Operation at any age is now safe with modern
     anaesthesia
(iv) Preoperative management
  a. Examine both sides and mark the appropriate side
  b. If for strangulation then sedate and place in gallows
     traction or over a pillow for one hour, if reduction
     then does not occur, proceed to surgery
 (v) Pre-incision
  a. General anaesthesia with optional endotracheal
     intubation
  b. Position
     Supine
  c. Skin preparation of lower abdomen and groins
(vi) Incision
  Groin skin crease incision above and parallel to medial
  inguinal ligament
(vii) Procedure (inguinal herniotomy)
  a. Divide superficial fascia
  b. Ligate and divide the superficial epigastric vein
  c. Locate the hernial sac at the external inguinal ring
     lying lateral to the cord/round ligament (the external
     ring overlies the deep ring in infancy)
  d. In an older child it may be necessary to open the
     inguinal canal by dividing the external oblique
     aponeurosis lateral to the external ring to gain
     access to the sac
  e. Very carefully dissect the covering layers of
     spermatic fascia and cremaster off the sac and
     gently separate the sac from the cord/round ligament
  f. The hernial sac may be completely into the scrotum
     and therefore contain the testis; if so, then carefully
     divide the sac at the top of the scrotum and pick up
     its proximal margins in forceps; otherwise open the
     apex of the sac. In both cases examine and reduce
     its contents to the abdomen
  g. In a strangulating hernia this should be done very
     gently as the mesentery of the small bowel and
     testicular vessels are easily damaged
  h. Transfix and ligate the neck of the empty sac with an
     absorbable suture. Excise any redundant sac

       i. Closure — Close the external oblique aponeurosis if opened

Close the superficial fascia as a separate layer

Close the skin with a subcuticular absorbable suture

(viii) Postoperative management
    a. Elective cases may be done as day-cases and sent home the same evening
    b. Emergency cases: await the return of normal bowel function

(ix) Complications
    a. Testicular infarction — Due to cord compression in strangulated hernias
    b. Recurrence — Due to incomplete excision of the sac

2. In adults
  (i) Principles
    a. More common in males (10:1 males:females)
    b. 90% indirect, 10% direct
    c. Operating for the second time in a male then it is wise to obtain consent for orchidectomy; such circumstances are usually exceptional
    d. Exclude any predisposing factors — Chronic obstructive airways disease
Bladder outflow obstruction
    e. Many operations and modifications have been described for this procedure, probably as testament to the fact that recurrence occurs with all, usually with an incidence of 5%.

  (ii) Preoperative management
    a. Examine both sides and mark the appropriate side
    b. Chronic obstructive airways disease may well need preoperative chest physiotherapy (or consider local anaesthetic, see page 10)
    c. If strangulating — Then needs resuscitation
Cross-match 2 units of blood
Broad spectrum and metronidazole antibiotic prophylaxis
Nasogastric aspiration
Catheterise

  (iii) Pre incision
    a. General anaesthesia with or without endotracheal intubation (essential in strangulation) or local anaesthetic infiltration (60 ml of 0.5% Marcaine)

b. Position
Supine
c. Skin preparation — All of abdomen and groin (if
laparotomy necessary)
(iv) Incision
Groin incision 3 cm above and parallel to the medial
two-thirds of the inguinal ligament
(v) Procedure
a. Ligate and divide the superficial epigastric vein
b. Locate the spermatic cord/round ligament as it
emerges at the external ring, divide the external
oblique aponeurosis laterally from the external ring
in the line of its fibres to expose the inguinal canal
c. Indirect hernia — Lies in front of the cord
Dissect the cremaster off the sac
and dissect the sac and cord apart
Open the apex of the sac, inspect
and reduce the contents
Transfix the sac at the deep ring
and excise the redundant sac
d. Direct hernia — Lies behind the cord in
Hasselbach's triangle
reduce the sac en-masse, unless
large, then open, reduce the
contents, transfix the neck and
excise the redundant sac
(vi) Strangulating hernia
a. Almost always indirect
b. Open the sac and assess the viability of the contents
c. If the contents have reduced spontaneously to the
abdomen, the constriction was probably minimal and
they are probably viable; therefore manage as an
indirect hernia. Examine the patient regularly postoperatively for evidence of obstruction or peritonitis
suggestive of necrotic bowel warranting a
laparotomy
d. If the contents look potentially viable, then gently
dilate the neck (agent of strangulation), increase the
patient's oxygenation and wrap the bowel in warm
saline soaked packs and reassess its viability after 10
minutes. If viable then return to the abdomen (good
colour, pulsatile mesenteric vessels). If it is not
viable or is of doubtful viability, then resect the
segment reconstituting the bowel with an end-to-end
anastomosis
(vii) In all cases perform a herniorraphy to reinforce the
posterior wall of the inguinal canal
Commence a nylon darn on the periostium of the

pubic tubercle, and loosely darn laterally taking alternate pieces of inguinal ligament and conjoint tendon/internal oblique muscle at 0.5 cm intervals as far as the deep ring, reducing the deep ring to admit only the cord, then return the darn in a similar fashion to the pubic tubercle. Complete the darn by tying the two ends together. Although there is no tension in the darn, this produces a strong repair of the posterior wall which has become weakened in indirect hernia and defective in direct hernia. This will excite fibrosis which will reinforce the repair.

(viii) Closure
  a. Repair the external oblique aponeurosis with an absorbable suture
  b. For a repeat repair in which the tissues may ooze then it may be wise to place a suction drain for 24 hours postoperatively
  c. Close in layers

(ix) Postoperative management
  a. Mobilise early; if young and fit may be done as 'day-case' surgery
  b. If strangulated, then commence oral fluids once the nasogastric aspirate is minimal and flatus has been passed per rectum

(x) Complications
  a. Hernia recurrence — 5%
  b. Strangulated hernia — Wound infection

Anastomosis — Leakage
              Stricture
Ileus

FEMORAL HERNIA: LOW REPAIR

1. Principles
   (i) Extremely rare in children
   (ii) Occurs more frequently in women than men, but even so, inguinal hernia is more common than femoral in women
2. Indications for surgery
   All femoral hernias
3. Preoperative management
   (i) Examine both sides and mark the appropriate side
   (ii) If strangulated
       a. Resuscitate and rehydrate
       b. Nasogastric aspiration
       c. Catheterise (empty the bladder as this may well be involved in the hernia)

        d. Cross-match 2 units of blood
        e. Broad spectrum and metronidazole antibiotic
          prophylaxis
4. Pre-incision
    (i) General anaesthesia and endotracheal intubation
       (possible to perform elective repair under local
       anaesthetic)
    (ii) Position supine
    (iii) Skin preparation of groin and abdomen for laparotomy
       if necessary (see page 100)
5. Incision
    6 cm long over medial inguinal ligament
6. Procedure
    (i) Divide superficial fascia in the line of the incision
    (ii) Identify the sac as it descends through the femoral canal
       medial to the femoral vein
    (iii) Beware
       a. Femoral vein — Laterally
       b. Long saphenous vein entering the femoral vein from
         its medial side 2 cm below the inguinal ligament
    (iv) Open the apex of the sac, identify and reduce the
       contents
    (v) Transfix the neck of the sac and excise any redundant
       sac
    (vi) Repair the femoral canal with three interrupted non-
       absorbable monofilament sutures from the pectineal
       ligament to the inguinal ligament
7. Strangulated hernia
    (i) Open the sac as for an elective hernia and send some of
       the fluid from the sac for microbiological examination
    (ii) Inspect the contents
    (iii) Gently digitally dilate the femoral canal (Hay-Groves
       maneouvre of dividing the lacunar ligament with the
       rare risk of bleeding from an aberrant obturator artery is
       rarely necessary)
    (iv) If possible gently draw down the strangulated contents
       of the sac, removing the agent of constriction and
       assess the contents. Increase the patient's oxygenation
       and wrap the bowel in warm saline soaked packs; if
       viable then return to the abdomen and repair the hernia
    (v) If the bowel is not viable but can be drawn down into
       the wound, then resect and repair with an end-to-end
       anastomosis. Return the bowel to the abdomen and
       repair the hernia
    (vi) If it is not possible to deliver the bowel for resection,
       then perform a low laparotomy (midline or paramedian
       incision) and reduce the bowel gently from the inside. If
       the bowel is perforated then place soft bowel clamps on

the proximal and distal bowel within the abdomen
before performing the maneouvre. If the bowel is not
viable, then perform the resection and anastomosis via
the abdominal incision (see laparotomy for bowel
obstruction, page 100)
    (vii) Repair the femoral hernia and close both wounds
 8. Closure
    (i) Approximate the deep tissues with absorbable sutures
    (ii) Close the skin
    (iii) No drains
 9. Postoperative management
    (i) As most of these patients are elderly, then day-case
         surgery is impractical
    (ii) Strangulated hernia — commence oral fluids once the
          nasogastric aspirate is minimal and flatus is passed per
          rectum
10. Complications
    (i) Recurrent hernia
    (ii) Strangulated
         a. Wound infection (usually by organisms isolated from
            fluid in the sac)
         b. Ileus
         c. Anastomosis —   Leakage
                            Stricture
         d. Perforation of bladder, especially if not catheterised
         e. Damage to femoral vein

INCISIONAL HERNIA

 1. Preoperative management
    (i) Full assessment of aetiological factors, especially chronic
         obstructive airways disease which both exacerbates the
         hernia and may be severely embarrassed by the return
         of a large amount of gut to the abdomen by surgical
         repair (see principles of prevention and treatment of
         pulmonary problems during operations, page 10)
    (ii) Would the patient cope better with an abdominal support
          and would the chances of successful repair improve with
          weight loss prior to surgery?
 2. Upper abdominal hernia
    (i) Empty the stomach with a nasogastric tube
 3. Pre-incision
    (i) General anaesthesia, endotracheal intubation and full
         muscle relaxation
    (ii) Position
          Supine
    (iii) Skin preparation of all abdomen
    (iv) Incision — Excise old scar

4. Procedure
    (i) Opening the peritoneum is a matter of personal preference and may be useful if combining the procedure with an intra-abdominal operation such as second look laparotomy in malignant disease
    (ii) Freshen and expose the free edges of the muscle or aponeurotic layers for about 3 cm lateral to the defect
    (iii) Close the defect with interrupted non-absorbable mattress sutures (Mayo repair) suturing one layer over the top of its counterpart)
5. Closure
    (i) A wound drain may be necessary if there is a significant ooze of blood from the tissues
    (ii) Close the superficial tissues in as many layers as can be constituted
6. Postoperative management
    Mobilise the patient as soon as possible; these patients are the same group who have a high incidence of DVTs and pulmonary problems, elderly and obese (see principles of prevention and treatment of DVT and pulmonary problems during operations, pages 7–11)
7. Complications
    (i) Wound infection
    (ii) Wound sinus from a non-absorbable suture
    (iii) Respiratory embarrassment
    (iv) Hernia recurrence

SIMPLE MASTECTOMY WITH AXILLARY SAMPLING

1. Preoperative management
    Examine and mark the side; full psychological support and advice about available prostheses. Shave axilla
2. Investigation
    (i) Diagnosis with needle biopsy/aspiration cytology ± oestrogen receptor status
    (ii) Mammography/xerography
    (iii) Isotope bone and liver scans for metastases
    (iv) Liver function tests for metastases
3. Pre-incision
    (i) Anaesthesia
        General anaesthesia with endotracheal intubation but possible under local anaesthetic if the patient is a poor anaesthetic risk
    (ii) Position
        Supine with the arm extended and supported on an arm board

    (iii) Skin preparation
        a. *Avoid iodine* since a hypersensitivity reaction may delay postoperative radiotherapy
        b. Pack the axilla with cotton wool
        c. Towel up to expose breast and axilla on affected side with the arm towelled separately and therefore mobile

4. Incision
Elliptical at least 2 cm above and below nipple and including the site of the tumour. The medial apex at the midline and the lateral apex beyond the anterior axillary line

5. Procedure
    (i) Elevate the upper skin flap by sharp dissection in the plane of the superficial fascia, medially as far as the sternum and laterally into the axilla. Raise this flap as far as the clavicular head of pectoralis major
    (ii) Elevate the lower skin flap as far as the inferior margin of breast tissue
    (iii) In both of these maneouvres dissection is aided by gentle counter traction on the breast and being careful to avoid button holing the skin
    (iv) Commencing medially, dissect the breast tissue off the deep fascia of pectoralis major ligating the perforating branches of the internal mammary vessels
    (v) As this dissection proceeds laterally *Beware*
        a. *Long thoracic nerve* on serratus anterior
        b. *Axillary vein* above the tail of the breast
    (vi) Remove the specimen for histological examination
    (vii) Explore the axilla to remove palpable lymph nodes behind lateral border of pectoralis major for histological examination

6. Closure
    (i) Absolute haemostasis is essential
    (ii) Place two suction drains, one medially and one laterally
    (iii) Close skin in a single layer with interrupted sutures (a large defect may need a split skin graft)
    (iv) Dress the wound with a support dressing for comfort

7. Postoperative management
    (i) Encourage early arm movement and test the function of the long thoracic nerve by assessing the ability of the patient to put her arm behind her head
    (ii) Full psychological support and measure for a prosthesis prior to discharge
    (iii) Remove the drains when dry and the sutures one week after surgery

8. Complications
   (i) Early
      a. Damage to long thoracic nerve
      b. Skin flap necrosis resulting in a defect which may
         need a split skin graft
      c. Psychological problems
   (ii) Late
      a. Local recurrence
      b. Effects of radiotherapy (dermatitis, pneumonitis,
         lymphoedema of arm)
      c. Metastatic disease

ADRENAL SURGERY

1. Indications for unilateral adrenalectomy
   (i) Phaeochromocytoma
   (ii) Cushings syndrome, due to cortical adenoma (20%) or
      carcinoma (2%)
   (iii) Conns syndrome due to cortical adenoma
2. Indications for bilateral total or subtotal adrenalectomy
   (i) Bilateral adrenal tumour
   (ii) Uncontrollable ACTH dependent Cushings syndrome
      (78%) (pituitary or ectopic)
   (iii) Advanced breast cancer (probably now redundant with
      the advent of steroid antagonist therapy: tamoxifen and
      aminoglutethamide)
3. Preoperative management
   (i) Adrenal localisation methods
      a. (IVP — now superceded by modern methods)
      b. Ultrasound
      c. Abdominal CT scanning
      d. MIBG scan for phaeochromocytoma
   (ii) Preparation
      a. Phaeochromo-   — α-Blockade with
         cytoma   phenoxybenzamine
                         (β-blockade only necessary if
                         the patient develops a
                         tachycardia)
                         Exclude multiple endocrine
                         neoplasia (2 and 3)
      b. Cushings syndrome— Large doses of corticosteroids
                         from the time that the tumour
                         or hyperplastic adrenal glands
                         are removed
      c. Prophylactic antibiotics in Cushings syndrome as the
         high circulating cortisol may diminish resistence to
         infection

    d. Control Cushings induced hyperglycaemia during surgery
    e. Central venous line and pressure monitor
    f. Arterial pressure line
    g. Swan-Gantz pulmonary wedge pressure monitor is useful for phaeochromocytoma surgery
    h. Nasogastric tube
    i. Urinary catheter
4. Pre-incision
  (i) General anaesthesia, endotracheal tube and cardiac monitor
  (ii) Position
    a. Bilateral approach — Supine
    b. Unilateral approach — Prone
  (iii) Skin preparation of all of exposed abdomen and trunk
5. Incision
  (i) Bilateral adrenalectomy and phaeochromocytoma — Extended midline or extended upper transverse
  (ii) Unilateral adrenalectomy — Paravertebral commencing 6 cm lateral to the spinous process of T10, descending to the 12th rib and following its line laterally to the posterior axillary line
6. Procedure
  (i) Anterior approach to the right adrenal
    a. Mobilise the right upper hemicolon and hepatic flexure medially
    b. Kocherise the duodenum
  (ii) Anterior approach to the left adrenal
    a. Mobilise the left upper hemicolon and splenic flexure medially
    b. Divide the splenorenal ligament and medially mobilise the spleen with tail of pancreas
  (iii) Posterior approach to the adrenal glands
    Via the bed of the 12th rib which is excised
  (iv) Beware opening the pleura (which may need to be closed over an underwater seal drainage system)
  (v) Specific points of adrenalectomy
    a. The adrenal gland is recognised by its golden yellow colour distinct from surrounding fat
    b. It receives at least three significant arterial supplies (the adrenal artery, the renal artery and phrenic artery)
    c. Left adrenal vein drains to the left renal vein
    d. Right adrenal vein is *very short and wide* and drains directly into the inferior vena cava; therefore inadvertent avulsion can be catastrophic

    (vi) Danger points of severe hypertension during
         adrenalectomy for phaeochromocytoma
         a. Induction of anaesthesia
         b. Lifting onto the operating table
         c. During handling of the adrenal gland
         d. Beware severe hypotension immediately after removal
            of the gland necessitating massive colloid transfusion
7. Postoperative management
     (i) Should be on an intensive care unit
    (ii) Phaeochromocytoma
         Regular cardiovascular monitoring with colloid
         replacement for hypotension
   (iii) Cushings syndrome
         Replacement corticosteroids initially in large doses and
         then slowly reduced over 4–6 weeks after surgery
         (initially parenterally and then orally)
    (iv) Commence oral fluids once nasogastric aspirate is
         minimal and flatus passed per rectum
8. Complications
     (i) Phaeochromocytoma
         a. Hypertensive crisis during surgery
         b. Hypotension after surgery
    (ii) Cushings syndrome — Addisonian crisis after surgery
   (iii) Ileus
    (iv) Wound infection
     (v) Late
         a. Phaeochromocytoma — Recurrent tumour in the
                                  other gland or sympathetic
                                  chain
                                  metastatic disease
         b. Cushings   — Hyperplasia of residual
                                  gland if resection is
                                  inadequate

LAPAROTOMY FOR PERITONITIS OF UNKNOWN CAUSE

1. Preoperative management
     (i) Resuscitation
         a. Intravenous fluids, especially colloids to restore the
            blood pressure
         b. Nasogastric aspiration
         c. Central venous pressure monitor
         d. Catheterise to monitor urine output
    (ii) Investigation
         a. Full blood count and electrolyte estimation
         b. Blood for microbiological culture

    c. Erect abdominal X-ray — Subphrenic gas
                              Obstruction
    d. ECG: exclude myocardial infarction as a cause of the pain
    e. Chest X-ray: exclude lower lobe pneumonia as a cause of the pain
    f. Urine microscopy
    g. Amylase to exclude pancreatitis
  (iii) Informed consent, warning of the possibility of a defunctioning colostomy if the peritonitis is due to colonic pathology
  (iv) Broad spectrum antibiotics and metronidazole for a full therapeutic course

2. Pre-incision
  (i) General anaesthesia with endotracheal intubation
  (ii) Position
     Supine
  (iii) Skin preparation of all of abdomen (nipples to thighs)
  (iv) Towel up to expose midline but able to extend incision to either xyphisternum or symphysis pubis

3. Incision
  (i) Peri-umbilical midline

4. Procedure
  (i) Pack off walls of wound with antiseptic soaked packs before opening the peritoneum
  (ii) Upon opening the peritoneum aspirate any free pus. Swab with a bacteriological throat swab and send this specimen for gram staining, culture and sensitivity
  (iii) Open the peritoneum for the length of the wound and suck out all the free fluid
  (iv) Gently perform a laparotomy to ascertain the cause (the smell of the gas released is usually indicative of the site; high gastrointestinal causes are initially odourless whereas colonic perforation smells faeculant)
  (v) Perform appropriate surgery (see relevant section)

5. Closure
  (i) Prior to closure, mop out the peritoneal cavity, including all its recesses and spaces for solid infected debris
  (ii) Gently irrigate the peritoneum with several litres of warm saline, continuously sucking this out to reduce the concentration of innoculating pathogenic organisms
  (iii) Close in layers

6. Controversies of management
  (i) Intraperitoneal lavage with topical antibiotics and antiseptics (eg. noxytyalin)
  (ii) Wound drainage
  (iii) Antiseptic wound irrigation

7. Postoperative management
   (i) Continue parenteral antibiotics for a full therapeutic course
   (ii) Commence oral fluids once the nasogastic aspirate is minimal and flatus is passed per rectum
8. Complications
   (i) Immediate
      a. Septicaemia
      b. Wound infection
      c. (Portal pyaemia)
   (ii) First month
      a. Intraperitoneal abscess
      b. Obstruction — Ileus
                        Adhesions
                        Anastomotic oedema
   (iii) Late
      a. Incisional hernia
      b. Obstruction — Adhesions
                        Anastomotic stricture

DRAINAGE OF AN INTRA-ABDOMINAL ABSCESS

1. Preoperative management
   (i) Establish the diagnosis
      a. Clinically, swinging pyrexia and malaise one week after abdominal surgery or trauma
      b. May be tender over the site of a collection
   (ii) Investigations
      a. Leucocytosis
      b. Raised alkaline phosphatase
      c. Chest X-ray may show gas filled subphrenic loculus with a fluid level
      d. Ultrasound localisation: allows aspiration of pus to confirm the diagnosis with microbiological examination and percutaneous drainage
      e. Indium labelled leucocyte scan (not widely available)
   (iii) Antibiotic prophylaxis (cephalosporin and metronidazole) to reduce the risk of septicaemia
   (iv) Operation is necessary as soon as the diagnosis is made
2. Pre-incision
   (i) General anaesthesia and endotracheal intubation
   (ii) Position — Supine, unless
      a. Posterior subphrenic — Lateral position
      b. Pelvic abscess — Lithotomy position
   (iii) Skin preparation of whole of abdomen
   (iv) Incision
      a. Over the site of the abscess
      b. Pelvic abscess, which is bulging into the anterior rectum; drain via the rectum

3. Procedure
   (i) The aim of drainage is to evacuate the pus, with
       minimal disturbance of the wall of the abscess in
       continuity with the peritoneum, therefore minimising
       intraperitoneal spillage
   (ii) Send pus for microbiological examination
   (iii) Gently digitally break down loculi
   (iv) Appendix abscess — Unless the appendix is obviously
        lying free within the abscess cavity and easily
        removable it should be left alone and removed
        electively 2–3 months later
   (v) Drainage — Place a large tube drain into the cavity and
       bring out through a separate incision (except rectally
       drained pelvic abscesses where this is impractial)
4. Closure
   (i) Irrigate the wound with antiseptic
   (ii) Close in layers with interrupted absorbable sutures
   (iii) Secure the drain with a stout suture
5. Postoperative management
   (i) Continue parenteral antibiotics until apyrexial
   (ii) Rectally drained pelvic abscess: needs daily rectal
        examination to prevent loculation of the cavity
   (iii) When the drainage is minimal and serous then
         gradually shorten the drain allowing the cavity to
         collapse
   (iv) If the drainage is persistent then consider a sinogram to
        exclude a fistula to the bowel
   (v) Culture any persistently purulent discharge
6. Complications
   (i) Early
       a. Septicaemia
       b. Fistula
       c. Wound infection
       d. Recurrent abscess
   (ii) Late
        a. Fistula
        b. Recurrent abscess
        c. Incisional hernia

Vascular surgery

PRINCIPLES OF ELECTIVE VASCULAR RECONSTRUCTION

1. Indications
   (i) Never risk life to save a limb
   (ii) Full preoperative workup must establish nature and extent of disease, showing a good run-in and good run-off
   (iii) Severe claudication < 200 m
   (iv) A sudden recent deterioration
   (v) Pathology is above the knee
   (vi) Claudication distance less than angina distance
2. Contraindications
   (i) Severe angina
   (ii) Systemic malignancy
   (iii) Recent myocardial infarction
   (iv) Pathology is below knee (poor run-off) except in limb salvage for critical ischaemia
3. Relative contraindications
   (i) Continuing smoking
4. Indications for amputation
   (i) Gangrene
   (ii) Severe rest pain not amenable to arterial reconstruction
   (iii) Uncontrollable infection, especially in diabetics
   (iv) Malignancy
5. Types of surgery
   (i) Arterial
       a. Endarterectomy
       b. Profundoplasty
       c. Bypass graft — Reverse or *in situ* vein
                          Synthetic
       d. Angioplasty — Dotter and Gruntzig percutaneous balloon (radiological)
                        Vein patch
                        Synthetic patch
   (ii) Sympathectomy
       a. Surgical
       b. Chemical

(iii) Endarterectomy
    a. Only for larger arteries which do not cross joints (eg aorta, iliacs and carotids)
    b. Problems — Subsequent initial deposition 1–2 mm thick
                 Distal intimal dissection
                 Extent of disease
(iv) Vein (by-pass graft/patch)
    a. Best material, available from long saphenous or cephalic veins
    b. Undergoes changes —
                 Narrows with subendothelial hypertrophy and intimal clot deposition
                 10% develop atheroma
                 Anastomotic stenosis
                 Fibrosis develops at valves and tributaries
(v) Synthetic
    a. Dacron — Very good replacement for large vessels (> 10 mm)
                 Knitted, easier to suture but needs leak proofing with unheparinised blood
                 Woven, more difficult to suture but requires minimal pre-clotting (More recent grafts have been developed with collagen impregnation which do not leak at all)

         Problems — Tend to buckle across joints
                 False aneurysms at anastomoses
                 Thick intimal deposition (2–4 mm)
                 Infection of implanted foreign material

    b. PTFE (Goretex) —
                 Useful for smaller arteries (eg superficial femoral)
                 Easy to suture and requires no pre-clotting
                 Problems, high 3-year failure rate (> 30%) compared with vein
                 Infection
                 Tendency to kink

    c. Human umbilical vein (Dardik) —
                 Difficult to handle, high early failure rate

6. Technical principles
    (i) Aim for a smooth flow by
        a. Avoiding loose flaps
        b. Avoiding both intrinsic and extrinsic constriction
        c. Avoid narrowing at anastomoses
    (ii) Handle all arteries and grafts with care
    (iii) Strict asepsis
    (iv) Preoperative antisepsis
    (v) Per and postoperative antibiotics
    (vi) Peroperative anticoagulation with heparin
7. Operations for aorto iliac disease
    (i) Aorto iliac endarterectomy
    (ii) Aorto femoral synthetic Dacron graft
    (iii) Femoro-femoral Dacron graft
    (iv) Axillo-femoral subcutaneous Dacron graft
8. Operations for femoropopliteal disease
    (i) Femoropopliteal bypass
        a. Reverse saphenous vein
        b. *In situ* saphenous veins
        c. PTFE (Goretex)
        d. Human umbilical vein (Dardik)
        e. Dacron
    (ii) Superficial femoral endarterectomy
    (iii) Profundoplasty
9. Operations for internal carotid disease
    (i) Endarterectomy
    (ii) Extracranial (superficial temporal) to intracranial (middle cerebral) anastomosis
10. Operations for coronary artery disease
    (i) Aorto coronary artery vein bypass graft
    (ii) Endarterectomy (short lesion in large artery)
    (iii) Internal mammary coronary anastomosis

AORTO-BIFEMORAL BYPASS GRAFT

1. Indications
    (i) Severe aorto iliac atherosclerosis
    (ii) Leriche syndrome
2. Preoperative preparation
    (i) Investigations to establish extent of disease
        a. Doppler pressure studies
        b. Arteriography
    (ii) Manage concomitant problems
        a. Stop smoking
        b. Control diabetes
        c. Control hypertension
    (iii) Antiseptic bath prior to surgery with swabs sent from the patient's skin and orifices to exclude foci of pathogenic organisms (especially *Staphylococcus aureus*)

(iv) Antibiotic prophylaxis
    a. Flucloxacillin or Cephalosporin for 2–5 days
(v) Tubes
    a. Catheterise, nasogastric tube and intravenous infusion
    b. Arterial line optional
3. Pre-incision
  (i) General anaesthesia with endotracheal intubation
  (ii) Position
    Supine with arms by the side
  (iii) Skin preparation from mid thorax to knees
  (iv) Incisions
    a. Longitudinal incisions over each common femoral artery at the groin (12 cm in length)
    b. Transverse abdominal (heals better and is less painful than a longitudinal incision)
4. Procedure
  (i) Assess patency of groin arteries
  (ii) Dissect out both common femoral arteries as they pass under the inguinal ligament to beyond their bifurcation
  (iii) Beware
    a. *Femoral vein, medially*
    b. *Femoral nerve, laterally*
    c. Avoid damage to groin lymph nodes
  (iv) Place silastic slings to control the common femoral, superficial femoral and profunda femoris arteries; smaller branches may also need slings
  (v) Full laparotomy to exclude other pathology
  (vi) Pack off small bowel
  (vii) Incise peritoneum to the left of the small bowel mesentery to approach the aorta
  (viii) Expose the aorta from the level of the left renal vein down to the bifurcation taking care to avoid and protect the inferior mesenteric artery
  (ix) Beware
    a. The vena cava on the right of the aorta
    b. The left common iliac vein behind the aortic bifurcation
  (x) Slings around the aorta at the upper and lower levels of dissection are optional (it may be necessary to mobilise both common iliac arteries and control these with slings if the aortic segment is short)
  (xi) Create tunnels behind the inguinal ligaments by blunt dissection
  (xii) Withdraw 20 ml of blood and preclot the graft
  (xiii) *Heparinise* the patient with 5,000 units either intravenously or directly into the aorta. *Wait three minutes*

(xiv) Now clamp across the aorta proximally and distally.
(xv) Clamp the common femoral arteries with appropriate clamps and their branches with bull-dog clamps
(xvi) Control lumbar arteries either from without or within by suture
(xvii) Open the aorta on its anterior surface; this may now require a local endarterectomy
(xviii) Cut the bifurcation graft to correct length with pre-bifurcation segment as short as possible to improve the haemodynamics of flow
(xix) Suture graft to aortic arteriotomy with continuous 3/0 prolene (either end-to-side or by aortic transection and end-to-end) and test the anastomosis by releasing the aortic clamp
(xx) Clamp the proximal graft and release the aortic clamps
(xxi) Pass sponge forceps from each groin wound through the predissected tunnels and withdraw the limbs of the graft to the groin wounds
(xxii) Open both common femoral arteries on their anterior surfaces just above their bifurcation. Avoid local endarterectomies
(xxiii) Anastomose one limb of the graft to the common femoral arteriotomies with 4/0 continuous prolene. The graft may be used as a patch to widen the orifice of the profunda
(xxiv) Release the clamps in turn to evacuate any clot which may have formed via the blow holes
(xxv) Establish flow in the completed limb
(xxvi) Suck out all the blood from the second limb and complete the second anastomosis
(xxvii) Release all the clamps and recheck the anastomoses
5. Closure
  (i) Once the ooze of blood from the graft and the anastomotic suture lines have subsided (heparin may occasionally require reversal with protamine) then commence closure
  (ii) No abdominal drains but suction drains to both groins
  (iii) Close the peritoneum over the graft in the abdomen to make it completely retroperitoneal and close the abdomen in layers
  (iv) Close the groins in layers
6. Postoperative management
  (i) Monitor peripheral pulses continuously and measure the arterial pressures in both legs by Doppler
  (ii) Continue antibiotics for five days

7. Complications
   (i) Early
      a. Anastomotic leakage uncommon
      b. Graft thrombosis is rare, needs re-exploration and thrombectomy (if this occurs there is usually poor run-in or run-off which must be dealt with)
      c. Graft infection
      d. Small bowel obstruction with adhesions to exposed graft if peritoneal cover is incomplete
      e. Lymphatic groin fistulae, usually heal spontaneously
   (ii) Late
      a. Aorto-enteric fistula
      b. Recurrent atheroma

REVERSE SAPHENOUS VEIN FEMOROPOPLITEAL BYPASS GRAFT

1. Indications
   Severe arterial insufficiency of the lower leg due to occlusion of the superficial femoral artery with poor collateral circulation between the profunda femoris and popliteal arteries
2. Preoperative preparation
   (i) Examine and mark out the vein with the patient standing
   (ii) Investigations to establish extent of disease
      a. Doppler pressure studies at rest and after exercise
      b. Arteriography
   (iii) Manage concomitant problems
      a. Stop smoking
      b. Control diabetes
      c. Control hypertension
   (iv) Antisepsis
      a. Shave the leg and antiseptic baths prior to surgery
      b. Preoperative and peroperative antibiotic prophylaxis with flucloxacillin continued for 2–5 days
      c. Mark out long saphenous vein with patient standing
   (v) IVI
3. Pre-incision
   (i) Either spinal or general anaesthesia with optional endotracheal intubation
   (ii) Position
       Supine with leg slightly flexed and abducted at the hip and the knee slightly flexed. Avoid compression of lateral popliteal nerve
   (iii) Skin preparation above groin to above ankle, whole leg
   (iv) Towel up to expose leg and place foot in a clear sterile bowel bag

4. Incision
   Groin incision 12 cm in length longitudinally over common
   femoral artery and a separate incision commencing distal to
   this over the length of the long saphenous vein to below the
   knee. The skin bridge between these two incisions improves
   lymphatic drainage from the leg
5. Procedure
   (i) Groin operator
       a. Dissect out the common femoral artery and its
          branches at the bifurcation. Place slings around the
          common femoral, profunda femoris and superficial
          femoral arteries (other larger branches if necessary)
       b. Dissect out the termination of long saphenous vein as
          it enters the femoral vein, ligate all its tributaries and
          its termination at the femoral vein. Divide the long
          saphenous vein 1–2 cm from its termination
       c. Dissect out the saphenous vein distally ligating and
          dividing all its branches as it passes under the skin
          bridge
   (ii) Lower operator
       a. Dissect out the lower popliteal artery dividing the
          deep fascia behind the saphenous vein, just below the
          knee
       b. Displace sartorius posteriorly or divide it near its
          insertion
       c. Bluntly dissect out the neurovascular bundle in the
          popliteal space as it passes between the heads of
          gastrocnemius (the medial head may be divided to
          improve access)
       d. Isolate the artery as it passes from medial to lateral
          behind the popliteal vein which is receiving the short
          saphenous vein, the tibial nerve lies laterally in the
          neurovascular bundle
       e. Place slings around the artery to control it
       f. Dissect out the long saphenous vein for the length of
          the incision, ligating and dividing all its tributaries. If
          the vein is inadequate, then use synthetic graft (eg
          PTFE)
       g. Now remove the long saphenous vein and turn it
          round, gently, inflate it with heparinised saline to test
          for leaks from tears and missed tributaries which must
          be closed
       h. *Heparinise the patient with 5,000 units* either
          intravenously or into the common femoral artery. *Wait
          three minutes*
       i. Clamp and control the femoral and popliteal arteries
          and all their local branches
       j. Open both arteries and if necessary perform a local
          endarterectomy of the common femoral artery

k. Replace the reversed vein subcutaneously and anastomose it firstly to the common femoral artery with a 5/0 prolene continuous suture side-to-end
l. Now anastomose the lower end of the vein graft to the popliteal artery end-to-side with a similar suture material, leaving a small blow-hole
m. Test the upper anastomosis by flushing through and out of the blow hole at the lower anastomosis. Allow any thrombus in the distal arteries out of the blow hole by backwards (retrograde) flow. Close the artery and remove the controlling clamps

6. Closure
   (i) Once the anastomotic suture line ooze has ceased and graft patency is established commence closure
   (ii) Place suction drains in groin wound and popliteal fossa
   (iii) Close deep fascia and skin separately

7. Postoperative management
   (i) Check pedal arterial pressures by Doppler regularly during recovery
   (ii) Nurse with leg slightly flexed at the knee and supported for 48 hours, mobilise after this
   (iii) Antibiotic cover for 48 hours

8. Complications
   (i) Graft occlusion
       a. Early — Usually due to technical error in surgery (can be reduced by peroperative angiography)
       b. Late — Recurrent disease either above, below or in graft, especially with continuing smoking
   (ii) Lymphatic leakage at groin
   (iii) Infection less serious with vein graft but increases the risk of secondary haemorrhage

PROFUNDOPLASTY

1. Indications
   (i) Thigh claudication due to profunda stenosis
   (ii) Lower leg ischaemia with profunda popliteal collateral circulation

2. Preoperative preparation
   (i) As for femoro popliteal bypass (see page 33)
   (ii) Investigations
       a. Lateral or oblique femoral arteriogram

3. Pre-incision
   As for femoro popliteal bypass (which may be necessary should profundoplasty not be feasible)

4. Incision
   Longitudinally for 12 cm over femoral pulse at groin

5. Procedure
    (i) Dissect out common femoral, superficial femoral and
        profunda femoris arteries in the femoral triangle
   (ii) Trace the profunda distally, ligating and dividing veins
        as they cross it, isolating its branches with slings
  (iii) Isolate and remove 5–6 cm of superficial vein. It is
        preferable to preserve the long saphenous vein for
        further arterial reconstruction
   (iv) Place slings around all the major arteries and
        heparinise the patient with 5000 units intravenously.
        Wait 5 minutes and clamp the major vessels at the
        edge of the operative field
    (v) Perform a long arteriotomy, commencing on the mid
        common femoral artery, passing down the profunda
        and finishing at its bifurcation or beyond if the vessel is
        still abnormal
   (vi) Perform a local endarterectomy for the length of the
        arteriotomy, suturing down the distal flaps of atheroma
        with non-absorbable sutures
  (vii) Close the arteriotomy with a long reversed vein patch
 (viii) Remove clamps to establish and check flow, await
        haemostasis at suture line
6. Closure
    (i) Suction drain to deep wound
   (ii) Close in layers
7. Postoperative management
    (i) As for femoro-popliteal bypass (see page 35) but can
        mobilise earlier

CAROTID ENDARTERECTOMY

1. Indications
    (i) Carotid stenosis with
        a. Unilateral transient ischaemic attacks or amaurosis
           fugax
        b. Mild persistent cerebrovascular defect
2. Relative indications
   Severe carotid stenosis (> 90%) without neurological deficit
3. Contraindications
    (i) Recent major stroke
   (ii) Asymptomatic carotid bruit with less than 75% stenosis
  (iii) Severely symptomatic abdominal aortic aneurysm
   (iv) Disseminated malignant disease
4. Relative contraindications
   Second side operation within two weeks of first side
5. Preoperative management
    (i) Investigation to establish diagnosis
        a. Duplex Doppler studies of carotids

         b. Arteriography
         c. CT scan of brain
     (ii) Aspirin is optional
    (iii) Examine and mark the side
6. Pre-incision
      (i) General anaesthesia with endotracheal intubation
     (ii) Position
          Supine with shoulders elevated on a pad to extend the
          neck and the head turned away
    (iii) Peroperative ECG
     (iv) Intravenous line and radial arterial line for continuous
          arterial pressure monitoring
      (v) Skin preparation from neck to thorax
     (vi) Drapes, expose from parotid area to root of neck
7. Incision
   Along anterior border of sterno-mastoid centering on the
   carotid bifurcation
8. Procedure
      (i) Divide platysma with the skin
     (ii) Retract greater auricular nerve posteriorly in upper part
          of wound and divide the deep fascia in the line of the
          incision
    (iii) Place a self retaining retractor to hold sternomastoid
          posteriorly, mobilise, ligate and divide the common
          facial vein to expose the carotid sheath
     (iv) Dissect the tissues of the carotid sheath off the
          carotids, exposing and preserving the hypoglossal
          nerve as it crosses the two carotids above the
          bifurcation of the common carotid artery
      (v) *Beware descendens hypoglossi and vagus nerve*
     (vi) Gently retract the hypoglossal nerve and descendens
          hypoglossi away from the arteries
    (vii) Gently pass slings around the common carotid, internal
          carotid and external carotid arteries
   (viii) *Beware rough handling causing embolisation of
          atheroma*
     (ix) *Heparinise with 5,000 units and wait three minutes*
      (x) Now gently occlude the carotids and start the stop
          watch which records carotid occlusion time, mobilise
          the common carotid bifurcation, clamping all major
          branches
     (xi) Measure the internal carotid stump pressure to
          determine whether a shunt is necessary
    (xii) A shunt is necessary if the internal carotid pressure is
          less than one-third of the radial artery pressure
   (xiii) Perform an arteriotomy at the site of the occlusion and
          if necessary pass a Javid shunt above and below the
          occlusion. Perform the endarterectomy

(xiv) Close the arteriotomy with 6/0 Prolene, removing the shunt at the end

(xv) Remove the clamps, first the external, then the common and finally the internal carotid, noting the clamped time on the stop watch

(xvi) Await haemostasis from suture line

9. Closure
   (i) Haemostasis, swab and instrument check
   (ii) Place suction drain in the wound
   (iii) Close in layers, deep fascia, and skin

10. Postoperative management
    Nurse in intensive care unit with quarter hourly observation of pulse, blood pressure and neurological observations.

11. Complications
    (i) Stroke (early) 2%; may be precipitated by hypotension
    (ii) Mortality < 2%

CERVICAL SYMPATHECTOMY — SUPRACLAVICULAR APPROACH

1. Indications
   (i) Hyperhydrosis of hand
   (ii) Raynaud's phenomenon
       a. Buerger's
       b. Polio
       c. Syringomyelia
   (iii) But little use in Raynaud's disease

2. Pre-operative preparation
   (i) Mark the side
   (ii) Warn the patient about the risk of Horner's syndrome and exclude pre-existing Horner's

3. Pre-incision
   (i) General anaesthesia with endotracheal intubation
   (ii) Position
       Supine with a sandbag under the shoulders and neck extended with head turned away

4. Incision
   (i) 8 cm long, 2 cm above and parallel to mid-third of clavicle

5. Procedure
   (i) Divide
       a. External jugular vein (beware air embolism)
       b. Lateral border of sternomastoid
       c. Omohyoid central tendon — marking the ends with ligatures
       d. Lateral scalenus anterior
   (ii) Beware phrenic nerve on scalenus anterior
   (iii) *Beware subclavian vein inferiorly, and thoracic duct on left* (if this is divided inadvertently, then ligate both free ends)

(iv) Insert torch on stick
(v) Place a sling around the subclavian artery, retracting it downwards
(vi) *Beware brachial plexus posteriorly*
(vii) Divide Sibson's fascia, depressing the dome of the diaphragm to palpate stellate ganglion on neck of first rib
(viii) Feel for and visualise the second and third thoracic sympathetic ganglia, which are to be removed
(ix) Remove these ganglia. Send the specimen for confirmatory histology
(x) *Beware opening pleura*
6. Closure
(i) If the pleura is inadvertently opened, reinflate the lung with positive pressure ventilation before closing
(ii) Suction drain in the floor of the wound
(iii) Repair
a. Omohyoid
b. Sternomastoid
(iv) Close in layers
7. Post-operative care
(i) Nurse sitting upright
(ii) Investigation
a. Chest X-ray in recovery, exclude pneumothorax
b. Histology of ganglia to confirm procedure
(iii) Complications
a. Horner's syndrome with T_1/stellate ganglion damage
b. Pneumothorax
c. Thoracic duct fistula, especially if damage to the thoracic duct is unrecognised at the time of surgery

LUMBAR SYMPATHECTOMY

1. Indications
Small vessel disease of the feet.
2. Pre-operative preparation
(i) If diabetic, test vibration sensations in the feet, since if absent, indicates that autonomic neuropathy also exists ∴ sympathectomy little use.
(ii) NG tube especially if bilateral since post-operative ileus is common.
3. Pre-incision
(i) General anaesthesia with endotracheal intubation.
(ii) Position
Supine with a sandbag under the lumbar region on the appropriate side.
(iii) Skin preparation of all of abdomen

4. Incision
   Transverse, lateral to umbilicus
5. Procedure
   (i) Deepen the incision through muscle layers with cutting
       diathermy as far as the peritoneum, *keep outside
       peritoneum*
   (ii) Mobilise posteriorly between peritoneum and
        transversus abdominis and gently work over psoas to its
        medial side
   (iii) Pack off retroperitoneal space with packs placed
         superiorly, inferiorly and medially, retracting the
         peritoneum and its contents medially with a large Deva
         retractor
   (iv) *Beware*
        a. *Ureter*
        b. *Gonadal vessels* } all travelling vertically
        c. *Aorta* on left
        d. *IVC* on right
        e. *Genito femoral nerve*
        f. Lumbar vessels
        g. Para-aortic lymph nodes (since they resemble
           sympathetic ganglia)
    (v) Identify sympathetic chain lying in groove between
        psoas and lumbar vertebral bodies visually and by
        palpation
   (vi) Lift chain with nerve hook and remove the second and
        third lumbar ganglia. Send for histological confirmation
6 Closure
   Close in layers
7 Post-operative management
   Complications
   a. Retroperitoneal haematoma
   b. Ileus especially if bilateral sympathetectomy
   c. Pain in distribution of the genito-femoral nerve

BELOW KNEE AMPUTATION FOR ISCHAEMIA

1. Pre-operative management
   (i) Examine and mark the side
   (ii) Special tests
       Is the case not suitable for arterial reconstruction?
       a. Dopplers
       b. Arteriogram
   (iii) Antibiotic
       a. Benzyl penicillin
       b. Metronidazole

2. Pre-incision
   (i) General or spinal anaesthesia
   (ii) No tourniquet
   (iii) Skin preparation
       a. Ankle to low abdomen (therefore possible to proceed to above knee amputation if necessary)
       b. Mark out skin flaps anterior: 10 cm below tibial condyle, posterior: 20 cm below tibial condyle
3. Incision
   Along line of skin flaps to deep fascia, ligate superficial veins
4. Procedure
   (i) Assess bleeding from skin edges. If poor, then probably not viable and consider above knee amputation
   (ii) Deepen incision in the anterior compartment dividing its muscles: tibialis anterior, extensor hallucis longus and extensor digitorum longus, ligate and divide the anterior tibial vessels
   (iii) Divide the tibia transversely at the level of the anterior flap and cut out an anterior bevel which should be filed until absolutely smooth and rounded and the filings washed out
   (iv) Divide the fibula with a Gigli saw 1–2 cm above the level of the division of the tibia
   (v) Divide the peroneal muscles at the same level as the fibula, ligating the peroneal vessels
   (vi) Ligate and divide the posterior tibial vessels then, with a sharp knife, divide the muscles of the deep compartment (tibialis posterior, flexor, digitorum longus and flexor hallucis longus) and the posterior compartment (soleus and gastrocnemius) between the posterior edge of the tibia and the posterior skin flap, ligating the deep veins of the calf
   (vii) Shave down the muscle of the posterior flap so that it lies comfortably opposing the anterior flap
5. Closure
   (i) Haemostasis must be meticulous
       a. Use ligatures
       b. *Avoid diathermy*
   (ii) Suction drain to raw muscle bed
   (iii) Suture
       a. Deep fascia of posterior flap to deep fascia and periostium of anterior flap with an absorbable suture
       b. Skin, interrupted monofilament sutures or steri strips
   (iv) Bandage stump
       a. Gauze
       b. Cotton wool
       c. Netalast

6. Postoperative management
    (i) Avoid any pressure, traditional stump bandaging is dangerous
    (ii) Keep knee in extension to reduce flexion contractures
    (iii) Encourage early exercises, especially with the patient prone for flexion and extension
    (iv) Commence walking training using an inflatable prosthesis
    (v) Attend fittings for prosthesis once wound healed
7. Complications
    (i) Early
        a. Infection (especially *Clostridium welchii*)
        b. Haematoma
        c. Skin flap ischaemia
    (ii) Late
        a. Stump — Neuroma
                     Osteoma
        b. Phantom limb (treat with carbimazipine)

ABOVE KNEE AMPUTATION FOR ISCHAEMIA

1. Pre-operative management
    (i) Special investigations
        a. Examine to assess level of ischaemia and mark the side
        b. Arterial Doppler pressures
        c. Arteriography
    (ii) Prophylaxis for *Clostridia* and coliforms for anus
        a. Penicillin
        b. Metronidazole
2. Pre-incision
    (i) General or spinal anaesthesia
        a. No tourniquet
    (ii) Skin preparation
        a. Low abdomen to upper shin with upper thigh to knee exposed
        b. Elevate knee with bowl to gain access posteriorly
        c. Mark out equal anterior and posterior skin flaps with medial and lateral apices 10 cm above the femoral condyles
3. Incision
    Along line of skin flaps to deep fascia, ligating superficial veins
4. Procedure
    (i) Assess skin flap bleeding for viability
    (ii) Deepen anterior flap through quadriceps femoris to femur, (ligate all major muscular vessels)
    (iii) Locate superficial femoral artery and vein in adductor canal; ligate and divide vessels separately

    (iv) Divide
       a. Adductors (magnus and longus)
       b. Sciatic nerve (ligate nutrient artery) and allow to
          retract
       c. Hamstrings (semimembranosus, semitendonosus and
          biceps femoris) posteriorly
       d. Ligating all bleeding muscular vessels
    (v) Place muscle guard on femur 10 cm above femoral
       condyles and divide femur at this point
   (vi) File femoral edges to remove sharp edges and wash out
       filings
5. Closure
    (i) Absolute haemostasis with ligatures (avoid diathermy)
   (ii) Swabs and instruments
  (iii) Suction drain to deep layers
  (iv) Loosely suture adductors to vastus lateralis over
      femoral stump
   (v) Suture superficial quadriceps to hamstrings with loose
      absorbable sutures
  (vi) Close deep fascia of anterior and posterior flaps
 (vii) Close skin
(viii) Bandage stump with
      a. Gauze
      b. Cotton wool
      c. Netalast
6. Post-operative management
    (i) Avoid traditional stump bandaging which is harmful
   (ii) If supine, place sandbags over stump to prevent flexion
      deformity with unopposed psoas flexion
  (iii) Commence stump exercises early
  (iv) Arrange limb fitting and mobilisation on stump when
      wound healed
7. Complications
    (i) Early
       a. Infection, especially *Clostridium welchii* and anaerobic
         coliforms
       b. Skin flap ischaemia
       c. Flexion contraction deformity
   (ii) Late
       a. Phantom limb
       b. Stump — Neuroma
                Osteoma

VARICOSE VEIN SURGERY

1. Indications
    (i) Venous ulceration
   (ii) Symptoms of venous stasis (itch, ache)

2. Contraindications
   Post phlebitic syndrome
3. Preoperative preparation
   (i) Assess varicosities
       a. To determine appropriate treatment
       b. To locate the site of all incompetent superficial to
          deep communications, especially sapheno-femoral
          incompetence
       c. Mark the site of all varicosities and incompetent
          perforating veins
   (ii) Investigations
       a. Doppler location of incompetent perforating veins
       b. Venogram, if leg is post phlebitic
4. Pre-incision
   (i) General anaesthesia is preferable to local anaesthesia
   (ii) Position
       a. Anterior veins, supine with legs apart
       b. Posterior veins, prone with legs apart
5. Incision
   (i) Groin, 4 cm in length in groin crease medial to femoral
       pulse
   (ii) Long saphenous strip, 3 cm longitudinally anterior to
        medial malleolus and groin incision
   (iii) Short saphenous ligation, 3 cm transverse in midline of
         popliteal fossa
   (iv) Perforating veins, 1–2 cm immediately over the site of
        the incompetent perforating vein
   (v) Stab avulsions, 2 mm stabs at site of avulsions
6. Procedure
   (i) Groin tie
       a. At the groin, dissect out the long saphenous vein as
          it enters the cribriform fascia, identifying all its
          tributaries, including the superficial epigastric,
          superficial pudendal and superficial external iliac
          veins
       b. Ligate and divide all these tributaries and the long
          saphenous vein as it enters the femoral vein (failure
          of surgery is usually due to a branch being missed
          and subsequently becoming varicose)
   (ii) Stripping
       a. Identify the long saphenous vein at the ankle and
          dissect out the sapheno femoral junction as for a
          groin tie operation
       b. Beware the saphenous nerve lying beside the vein at
          the ankle
       c. Open the vein at the ankle and pass the stripper
          proximally negotiating the venous tortuosities to the
          groin where the stripper head can be attached

d. Strip the vein from the groin to the ankle. This way reduces the chance of inadvertent damage to the saphenous nerve. Prior to stripping bandage the leg firmly from groin to ankle
(iii) Short saphenous vein
a. Ligate and divide it as it enters the deep fascia of the popliteal fossa (this may need an on-table venogram to determine its junction with the popliteal vein)
(iv) Incompetent perforating veins
a. Dissect out the varicosities over the perforating vein and ligate and divide all the branches, including the perforator as it enters the deep fascia
(v) Stab avulsions
a. Insert fine mosquito forceps through the stabs to pick up the underlying vein, gently withdrawing it. Apply gently tractions to avulse the vein and control bleeding with direct pressure
7. Closure
(i) Close skin except stab avulsions which need no closure
(ii) In every case, bandage the leg fully to the level of the highest vein
8. Postoperative management
Mobilise as soon as possible in support stockings

LEAKING ABDOMINAL AORTIC ANEURYSM

1. Pre-operative preparation
(i) Establish diagnosis
a. Clinically, reinforced by plain X-rays of abdomen including lateral view
b. Cross-match 8 units immediately
(ii) Transfer directly to the operating theatre and continue resuscitation in the anaesthetic room
(iii) Insert
a. At least two venous lines, including a central venous catheter
b. Catheter
c. NG tube ⎱ can possibly wait until
   arterial line ⎰ patient anaesthetised
(iv) Do not waste time trying to get the patient's blood pressure up prior to anaesthesia
(v) Antibiotics with induction
a. Broad spectrum
b. Flucloxacillin
(vi) No Heparin
2. Pre-incision
(i) Have the following instruments ready prior to making the incision

a. Aortic compressor to get control of the aorta with
compression through the lesser sac
b. 3 Foley urethral catheters with syringes ready to
inflate balloons
c. A selection of large vascular clamps such as
— Satinsky
De Bakey
CraaFoord
(ii) Place the conscious patient on the table, surgeon
on the right, paint abdomen with iodine in
alcohol and towel up for a long midline incision
(iii) Induce general anaesthesia and intubate
3. Procedure
(i) On induction perform a long midline incision (since the
tamponade effect of abdominal muscle tone is now
lost)
(ii) *Get control*
(iii) Pack small bowel up to the right
(iv) Small retroperitoneal leak
a. Dissect peritoneum off aorta and place clamps
across the neck and lower end of the sac
b. If you lose control during the procedure then incise
the sac and push your right thumb up into the neck.
Replace it with Foley catheter and inflate the balloon
to control bleeding
c. Place Foley catheters distally into both common iliac
arteries and underrun lumbar artery orifices with silk
(v) If there is a torrential intraperitoneal haemorrhage,
compress the aorta via the lesser sac with an aortic
compressor, suck out the peritoneum and then manage
as above
(vi) *Structures to beware in all these procedures*
a. Inferior vena cava to the right
b. Inferior mesenteric vein to the left
c. Left common iliac vein below aortic bifurcation
d. Left renal vein at the neck of the sac
(vii) Proceed
(viii) Incise sac longitudinally and semi-circumferentially at
its neck
(ix) Underrun orifices of lumbar and median sacral arteries
(x) Oversew orifice of the inferior mesenteric artery
(xi) Clean out organised clot within the sac, select graft
a. Tube/bifurcation
b. Size
c. Knitted versus woven Dacron
(xii) Insert graft with single continuous layer of
monofilament 3/0 Prolene suture, first at the top end
and then at the lower end

   (xiii) Prior to closure of lower end, check for back flow — if this is minimal then Fogarty catheter distally for emboli of fibrin and thrombus

   (xiv) Inspect sigmoid colon for ischaemia due to ligation of inferior mesenteric artery

   (xv) Close aneurysm sac over Dacron graft

4. Closure
   (i) Haemostasis
   (ii) Repair posterior peritoneum
   (iii) No drains
   (iv) Close peritoneum over graft to prevent adhesions between small bowel and the Dacron
   (v) Close abdomen in layers

5. Problems of procedure
   (i) Distal emboli, needs Fogarty embolectomy
   (ii) Aneurysm extends into iliac arteries then use aorto bifemoral bifurction graft with ligation of iliac aneurysms

6. Post-operative care
   Nursing
   a. ITU for 24 hours with half-hourly observation, especially — Pulse and BP
                              CVP
                              ECG
                              Feet — Pulses
                                        Temperature of skin
                              Urine output
   b. Check Hb and transfuse accordingly

7. Complications
   (i) Early
      a. Suture line leakage
      b. Bleeding as blood pressure rises after large transfusion
      c. Acute renal failure
      d. Myocardial infarction
      e. Acute sigmoid colon ischaemia
      f. Emboli to legs (trash foot)
   (ii) Late
      a. Other aneurysms, especially — Iliac
                                        Femoral
                                        Splenic
                                        Thoracic aorta
                                        Popliteal
      b. False aneurysm of graft especially at suture line
      c. Graft infection
      d. Aorto-duodenal fistula

FEMORAL EMBOLECTOMY

1. Pre-operative preparation
   (i) Mark side
   (ii) If the diagnosis is suspected
       a. Fully heparinise with 10,000 units i.v. as a bolus and continue as an infusion of 10,000 units 6 hourly
       b. Increase oxygenation
       c. Shave both groins so that both may be explored if necessary
2. Pre-incision
   (i) Anaesthetic
       a. If fit for general anaesthetic (GA), then GA with endotracheal intubation
       b. If not fit for GA — local anaesthetic (LA) infiltration of the groin with light sedation and analgesia
   (ii) Skin preparation of both groins, abdomen and thighs, exposing both groins
3. Incision
   Longitudinally over site of common femoral artery midway between symphysis pubis and anterior superior iliac spine
4. Procedure
   (i) Expose common, superficial and profunda femoral arteries
   (ii) Assess the presence of a pulse (if the embolus is lying at the bifurcation of common femoral, then a pulse is palpable proximally but not distally)
   (iii) Place silastic slings around vessels to control blood flow (clamps tend to break up and embolise thrombus and embolus)
   (iv) Perform arteriotomy at femoral bifurcation — remove blood clot/embolus and send for histological examination
   (v) Fogarty catheter
       a. Initially proximally with a large catheter to establish flow (always check balloon prior to use), then clamp
       b. Then distally down both main vessels to establish back flow with a smaller catheter, then clamp
   (vi) *Beware,* overinflation of Fogarty catheter balloon can damage vessel intima
5. Closure
   (i) Arteriotomy with 4/0 Prolene with a vein patch if the artery is narrow
   (ii) *Check distal pulses* once the arteriotomy is released
   (iii) Haemostasis
   (iv) Close in layers
   (v) If embolectomy is delayed then consider fasciotomy

6. Post-operative management
   (i) Palpate foot pulses regularly and measure pedal
       pressures by Doppler
   (ii) Continue to heparinise and subsequently warfarinise
   (iii) Investigate
       a. Histology of embolus
       b. Echocardiogram to exclude mural thrombus as source
          of embolism
       c. If echocardiogram negative then aortogram with
          lateral views
7. Complications
   (i) Prognosis if treated within 12 hours 80% successful
   (ii) If treated later than 12 hours, 20% successful
   (iii) Recurrent thrombosis, especially if acute ischaemia was
         due to thrombosis on ulcerated atheroma rather than
         embolism
   (iv) Lymphatic groin fistula/leakage
   (v) Compartment syndrome if embolectomy delayed

SADDLE EMBOLUS

The same approach is adopted, the exception being that bilateral
femoral control is necessary. It is usually possible to remove the
embolus intact from one groin with a Fogarty catheter. Access to
the other femoral artery is useful if embolectomy on the first side
fails and also if the procedure produces subsequent embolism
down the other side

Head and neck surgery

SUPERFICIAL PAROTIDECTOMY

1. Preoperative management
   (i) Examine the patient and mark the side, explain risk to VIIth nerve and exclude any prior VIIth nerve weakness
2. Investigation
   (i) Group and save
   (ii) Plain X-ray of parotid region
   (iii) Sialogram (stone disease, may show tumour in deep lobe)
3. Special preparation
   Shave side of face to temple
4. Pre-incision
   (i) Anaesthesia
      a. General with endotracheal intubation
      b. Avoid long acting muscle relaxants as they render the nerve stimulator ineffectual especially when seeking the smaller divisions of the facial nerve
   (ii) Position
      a. Supine with head supported and tilted slightly away from affected side
      b. A slight head up tilt on the table relieves venous congestion
   (iii) Preparation
      a. Towel up with the whole of the face exposed, or drape the face in translucent plastic allowing assessment of stimulation of all branches of VIIth during dissection
5. Incision
   Pre-auricular extending under ear and down anterior border of sternomastoid
6. Procedure
   (i) Elevate the skin flap anteriorly with skin hooks and locate the origin of the VIIth nerve lying anterior to the mastoid process; inferior to the bony external auditory meatus, emerging from the stylo mastoid foramen and lateral to styloid process

   a. NB: it lies 1 cm medio-inferiorly to the pointed end of the trigonal cartilage of the ear
   b. The trunk lies deep to the finger nail of an index finger placed with the distal inter phalangeal joint on the mastoid process (Beahrs)
   c. The main trunk bisects an angle between posterior belly of digastric and the bony tympanic plate
   d. Its position can be elicited by use of a nerve stimulator, watching the effects of stimulation on the facial muscle groups (especially useful for the smaller divisions)
   (ii) Locate the preserve greater auricular nerve for use if nerve grafting of the facial nerve is necessary
   (iii) Since the VIIth nerve becomes very superficial anteriorly never elevate the anterior skin flap further than the dissection of the parotid gland
   (iv) Dissect superficial parotid from deep parotid in the plane of the facial nerve
   (v) If the tumour involves the nerve then the central divisions may be sacrificed since they have good anastomoses, but superior and inferior division should be replaced by nerve graft if it is necessary to excise them
   (vi) Structures to beware
      a. VIIth nerve
      b. Parotid duct
      c. External carotid artery and retromandibular vein deep to VIIth nerve
   (vii) Remove the specimen after ligation and division of the parotid duct
7. Closure
   (i) Absolute haemostasis
   (ii) Suction drain to wound
   (iii) Oppose edges with several subcutaneous sutures and close skin with interrupted fine monofilament sutures
8. Post-operative management
   Remove
   a. Drain when dry, 24 hours
   b. Sutures, 2–3 days
9. Investigations
   Histology of specimen
10. Complications
   (i) VIIth nerve damage, usually neuropraxia. If permanent then consider
      a. Hypoglossal hitch
      b. Nerve graft with greater auricular nerve donor
      c. Plastic surgery
   (iii) Fistula, usually closes spontaneously; if persists then treat with radiotherapy

    (iv) Frey's syndrome, due to disorganisation of post-
         ganglionic sympathetic fibres and pre-ganglionic
         parasympathetic fibres. Treatment: divide greater
         superficial petrosal nerve carrying preganglionic
         parasympathetic fibres (tympanic neurectomy)

EXCISION OF SUBMANDIBULAR GLAND

1. Pre-operative management
   - (i) Examine and mark the side
   - (ii) Assess
     - a. Hypoglossal nerve
     - b. Mandibular branch of facial nerve
     - c. Lingual nerve
   - (iii) Shave chin and neck
2. Special investigations
   - (i) Sialogram
   - (ii) Plain X-rays of floor of mouth
3. Pre-incision
   - (i) Anaesthesia
     - a. General anaesthesia with endotracheal intubation
   - (ii) Position
     Supine, with head supported on a ring, extended on
     neck and turned away
   - (iii) Skin preparation from mouth to lower neck with separate
     head towel
   - (iv) Expose face and lower mouth
4. Incision
   Parallel and at least 2 cm below line of posterior third of
   mandible, *thus avoiding mandibular branch of facial nerve*
5. Procedure
   - (i) Divide platysma and deep cervical fascia in the line of
     the incision to expose the lower pole of gland and
     dissect it free
   - (ii) Retract posteriorly
     Posterior belly of digastric and stylohyoid
   - (iii) Doubly ligate and divide the facial artery as it enters
     the posterior operative field
   - (iv) Retract mylohyoid, exposing the deep part of the gland
   - (v) Dissect out the deep gland
   - (vi) *Beware*
     a. *Hypoglossal nerve* } lying on hyoglossus deep to the
     b. *Lingual nerve* } pole of the gland
   - (vii) *Ligate and divide Wharton's duct — protect lingual
     nerve passing anteriorly underneath from lateral to
     medial*
   - (viii) Remove gland

6. Closure
   (i) Meticulous haemostasis
   (ii) Suction drain to wound
   (iii) Close in layers
7. Post-operative management
   Remove
   a. Suction drain when dry
   b. Sutures at 3–5 days
8. Special investigation
   Histology of gland
9. Complications
   (i) Nerve damage
      a. Mandibular branch of VIIth nerve
      b. Hypoglossal nerve
      c. Lingual nerve
   (ii) Infection
   (iii) Submandibular fistula is very uncommon

EXCISION OF A STONE IN THE SUBMANDIBULAR DUCT

1. Indications
   (i) Impaction of a calculus at or near the orifice of the submandibular duct
   (ii) Posterior duct stones should be treated by excision of the submandibular gland (see page 52)
2. Preoperative management
   (i) Investigations
      Plain X-ray of the floor of the mouth
   (ii) Broad spectrum antibiotics if concomittant submandibular sialoadenitis
   (iii) IVI
3. Pre-incision
   (i) General anaesthesia with nasotracheal intubation and pharyngeal pack
   (ii) Position
      a. Supine with head supported
      b. Mouth kept open with self retaining retractor
4. Procedure
   (i) Palpate the stone gently, avoid pushing it backwards into the gland. *Impalpable stone: do not proceed*
   (ii) Retract the tongue to the opposite side
   (iii) Pass a catgut suture under the duct behind the stone to prevent it slipping backwards
   (iv) Pass a similar suture under the duct immediately in front of the stone
   (v) *Beware passing the sutures too deeply as the lingual nerve is passing under duct*

(vi) Incise the duct directly over the calculus and lift the stone out of the duct
5. Closure
  (i) Haemostasis
  (ii) Do not close opening in duct
  (iii) Remove pharyngeal pack
6. Post operative management
  Culture any pus exuding from duct
7. Complications
  (i) Early
    a. Sialoadenitis
    b. Reactionary haemorrhage
  (ii) Late
    a. Recurrent stone
    b. Consider exicision of submandibular gland (see page 52)

TRACHEOSTOMY

1. Indications
  (i) Improve ventillation
  (ii) Relieve obstructed airway
  (iii) Radical head and neck surgery
  (iv) Assist bronchial toilet, respiratory care
2. Pre-operative management
  (i) Investigations
    a. Respiratory function tests: blood gases
    b. Chest X-ray
  (i) Shave neck
  (ii) Antibiotics
    If indicated as a result of microbiological results from sputum
  (iii) Endotracheal tube may already be *in situ*
  (iv) IVI
  (v) Catheter/NG tube usually already in situ because of requirements for tracheostomy
3. Pre-incision
  (i) Anaesthesia, either
    a. Local (infiltrate 1% lignocaine with 1:300,000 adrenaline)
    b. General
  (ii) Position
    Supine, shoulders elevated on a sandbag with the neck extended
  (iii) *Check proposed tube: size and cuff function*
  (iv) Towel up, paint mouth to nipple with head towelled in separate head towel

4. Incision
   (i) Elective
      Transverse 2 cm above sternal notch — 5 cm long
   (ii) Emergency
      a. Vertical immediately above sternal notch
      b. Consider crico thyroid stab
   (iii) *Beware*, in babies the innominate vein may lie *above* the sternal notch
5. Procedure
   (i) Deepen incision through platysma and deep cervical fascia
   (ii) Open the strap muscle longitudinally in the midline
   (iii) Divide the thyroid isthmus between haemostats and oversew the free edges with an absorbable suture to maintain haemostasis
   (iv) If performed under local anaesthetic, inject trachea directly and spray mucosa with 2 ml of 1% lignocaine to depress the cough reflex
   (v) Open trachea
      a. Lift up cricoid cartilage with hook
      b. Cut out disc of 3rd ring 1 cm in width or create a Bjork flap based on the 4th tracheal ring
      c. Visualise endotracheal tube
   (vi) Remove endotracheal tube, insert tracheostomy tube and obturator, remove obturator and attach the tracheostomy tube to the ventillator
   (vii) Secure the tube with ties
6. Closure
   (i) Absolute haemostasis
   (ii) No drain
   (iii) Close very loosely in layers around the tracheostomy tube
7. Post-operative management
   (i) Half-hourly observation until stable on intensive care unit
   (ii) At bedside
      a. Humidifier
      b. Oxygen for tracheostomy tube
      c. Suction
      d. Dressing pack
      e. Retractor
      f. Tracheal dilator
      g. Good overhead light
8. Investigation
   (i) Chest X-ray
      a. Position of tube
      b. Exclude pneumothorax/surgical emphysema
   (ii) Blood gases
   (iii) Remove sutures, 5–7 days

(iv) If breathing spontaneously consider changing tube to a silver speaking type
9. Complications
    (i) Early
        a. Surgical emphysema, especially in the mediastinum
        b. Pneumothorax
        c. Tube — Obstruction
                     Displacement
        d. Tracheal/tube encrustation
        e. Haemorrhage — Reactionary
                           Secondary
    (ii) Late
        a. Tracheal stenosis
        b. Tracheo-cutaneous fistula

SUBTOTAL THYROIDECTOMY

1. Pre-operative management
    (i) Warn patient of the incidence of postoperative hypothyroidism and recurrent hyperthyroidism in Graves disease
    (ii) Special investigations
        a. Thyroid — Thyroid function test and antibodies
                       Isotope uptake scans
                       Plasma calcium level
                       Indirect laryngoscopy to
                           check cords
        b. Blood group and save
    (iii) Special preparation
        a. If hyperthyroid then render as euthyroid as possible pre-operatively with carbimazole and propranolol and continue propranolol for at least 10 days postoperatively
        b. Lugols iodine for two weeks preoperatively reduces the vascularity of the gland
    (iv) IVI
2. Pre-incision
    (i) Anaesthesia
    general anaesthesia with endotracheal intubation
    (ii) Position
    Supine with shoulders supported on a sandbag and neck extended. Support head on a ring. 5° head up tilt of operating table reduces venous engorgement
    (iii) Surgeon on side opposite lobe to be operated upon
    (iv) Skin preparation, towel up to expose the whole of the anterior neck
    (v) Skin, impress line of incision 3 cm above sternal notch with stout silk

3. Incision
   Incise skin and platysma together in a collar incision 8 cm in length
4. Procedure
   (i) Elevate flaps of skin with platysma
     a. Superiorly to thyroid cartilage
     b. Inferiorly to suprasternal notch
     c. Place Joll's retractor to retract skin flaps
   (ii) Divide
     a. Deep cervical fascia longitudinally in the midline
   (iii) Separate strap muscles and retract laterally
   (iv) Assess goitre
   (v) Ligate and divide in continuity
     a. Middle thyroid vein
     b. Superior thyroid vessels at the upper pole of the thyroid
   (vi) *Beware external laryngeal nerve*
   (vii) *Identify and beware recurrent laryngeal nerve* as it enters the operative field from below
   (viii) Ligate and divide the branches of the inferior thyroid artery on the capsule of the gland (division laterally can embarrass the blood supply of the parathyroids)
   (ix) Divide isthmus and place haemostats around margin of resection leaving 2 g of thyroid from each lobe
   (x) *Identify and beware parathyroids*
   (xi) Any doubt as to whether yellow tissue is parathyroid or fat, use the density test by placing in a jar of water. Parathyroid tissue will sink slowly whereas fat will float on the surface
   (xii) Repeat partial lobectomy on opposite side
5. Closure
   (i) Absolute haemostasis
   (ii) Suction drain to thyroid bed
   (iii) Close loosely in layers with absorbable sutures
   (iv) Close the skin with sutures or clips
   (v) *Check vocal cords on extubation by direct laryngoscopy*
6. Post-operative management
   Nursing
   a. Half-hourly observation till conscious
   b. At bed side — Michel clip remover in case of respiratory distress due to haematoma
                     10 ml calcium gluconate 10% in case of acute hypocalcaemia
   c. Keep semi recumbant
7. Investigations
   (i) Review indirect laryngoscopy (especially if there is cord impairment on extubation)
   (ii) Serum calcium regularly postoperatively

(iii) Thyroid function tests at 6 weeks postoperatively
(iv) Remove
  a. Drain when dry, 24–48 hours postoperatively
  b. Sutures/clips, 2–3 days postoperatively
8. Complications
  (i) Early
    a. Haemorrhage, usually reactionary
    b. Tetany — In first three days from corrected
       thyrotoxicosis
       After one week with hypoparathyroidism
    c. Recurrent laryngeal nerve palsy — 95% neurapraxia
       and resolves
       If bilateral . . .
       cords *adduct* to
       midline
       *So needs
       immediate re-
       intubation*
    d. Thyroid crisis, if thyrotoxic patient is inadequately
       prepared, rare with modern techniques
  (ii) Late
    a. Keloid scar
    b. Hypothyroidism — 20% of all patients undergoing
       partial thyroidectomy
    c. Recurrent thyrotoxicosis, < 5% of patients undergoing
       thyroidectomy for Graves disease

PRINCIPLES OF PARATHYROID SURGERY

1. Preoperative management of hyperparathyroidism
  (i) Reduce calcium intake, 500 mg daily calcium diet
  (ii) Rehydrate orally or intravenously if severely
       hypercalcaemic (NB steroids have no place in the
       management of hyperparathyroidism)
  (iii) *Exclude associated pathologies*
    a. Those due to hypercalaemia
       Urinary tract stones
       Duodenal ulcer
       Pancreatitis
       Psychosis
    b. Those associated with hyperparathyroidism chronic
       renal failure
    c. Those associated with parathyroid hyperplasia
       Multiple endocrine neoplasia Type II
       Medullary carcinoma thyroid
       Phaeochromocytoma

d. Those associated with parathyroid adenoma
   Multiple endocrine neoplasia Type I
   Pancreatic endocrine tumours
   Pituitary tumours
2. Parathyroid localisation studies

Method	Accuracy
Ultrasound (with aspiration cytology)	50–80% tumours of > 0.5 cm
CT	> 70% of tumours > 1.0 cm
Angiography — PTH venous sampling	Only lateralising
Selective arteriography	80%
Subtraction technetium thallium isotope scan	90%

   (i) Other tests
       a. Group and save
       b. Indirect laryngoscopy to assess vocal cords
3. Neck exploration
   (i) As for thyroidectomy (see page 56)
   (ii) Mobilise the thyroid by ligation and division of the
        middle thyroid veins
   (iii) Fully explore both sides and account for all the
         parathyroids
4. Peroperative methods of parathyroid localisation
   (i) Methylene blue method, turns patient blue
   (ii) Wang's density test, accurately differentiates adenomata
        from hyperplasia
   (iii) Frozen section examination, needs an experienced
         parathyroid pathologist
5. Problems of parathyroid surgery
   (i) Localisation of all four glands
   (ii) Common sites of ectopic glands
       a. Within the carotid sheath
       b. Retropharyngeal
       c. Within the thymus
       d. Within the thyroid (usually enveloped by a
          multinodular goitre)
       e. Superior mediastinum
   (iii) Management of single versus multiple gland disease
       a. Single adenoma, excise
       b. Multiple adenoma, excise, leaving normal glands
       c. Hyperplasia, either excise 3½ glands or total
          parathyroidectomy with forearm reimplantation of
          100 mg of parathyroid tissue

6. Closure
As for thyroidectomy (see page 57)
7. Postoperative management
   (i) Nurse semi recumbant and prepared to remove sutures at the first sign of respiratory embarrassment due to haematoma collection
   (ii) Investigation
      a. Daily calcium estimation [if hypocalcaemic then correct with 1-α-calcidol (vitamin D) and oral or parenteral calcium]
      b. Histology of parathyroids
      c. Indirect laryngoscopy of vocal cords
8. Complications
   (i) Recurrent laryngeal nerve damage (as with thyroidectomy, see page 58)
   (ii) Hungry bone disease causing profound hypocalcaemia — rare, usually associated with parathyroid bone disease
   (iii) Recurrent hypercalcaemia
      a. Inadequate excision or missed adenoma
      b. Other cause of hypercalcaemia (malignancy, sarcoid etc)

THYROGLOSSAL CYST AND FISTULA

1. Preoperative management
   Special investigations, ultrasound of the neck
2. Pre-incision
   (i) General anaesthestic preferably with nasotracheal intubation
   (ii) Position and skin preparation — as for thyroidectomy (see page 56)
3. Incision
   (i) Cyst, transverse over cyst
   (ii) Fistula, transverse elliptical around fistula opening
4. Procedure
   (i) Cyst
      a. Divide platysma in the line of the incision
      b. Divide the deep cervical fascia and strap muscle longitudinally in the midline over the cyst
      c. Excise the cyst
      d. Dissect out any fibrous track towards the hyoid bone as for a fistula (see below)
   (ii) Fistula
      a. Sharply dissect out ascending fistula track as it passes between the strap muscles
      b. Elevate the upper skin flap with platysma to assist the dissection

    c. Follow the fistula track up to the hyoid bone to which it is intimately related

    d. Gently mobilise the body of the hyoid bone from its muscular attachment (mylohyoid, sternohyoid and thyrohyoid)

    e. Excise the centre part of the body of hyoid *en bloc* with the fistula track

    f. Follow and excise any remnant of the fistula track by dividing the median raphe of mylohyoid (it may continue as far as the foramen caecum of the tongue)

    g. The final procedure can be aided by the assistant depressing the posterior tongue with his index finger

5. Closure
   (i) Absolute haemostasis
   (ii) Suction drainage
   (iii) Close in layers

6. Postoperative management
   (i) Remove the drain on the first postoperative day and sutures after 72 hours
   (ii) Investigations, histological examination of the specimen

7. Complications
   Recurrence of the fistula if inadequately excised or in the case of a thyroglossal abscess treated by simple drainage

EXCISION OF BRANCHIAL FISTULA

1. Preoperative management
   (i) Examine and exclude the presence of *Bilateral* fistulae.
   (ii) Warn the patient that the procedure may need several incisions
   (iii) Investigations
       a. Lipiodol sinogram of track is optional
       b. Aspiration of branchial cyst shows cholesterol crystals on microscopy

2. Pre-incision
   (i) General anaesthesia with endotracheal intubation
   (ii) Position
       Supine with the neck extended and the head turned slightly away
   (iii) Skin preparation of lower face to upper chest
   (iv) Towel up head separately and expose the whole of the lower face and neck on the affected side
   (v) Prior to incision, inject 3–5 ml of methylene blue into the fistula opening to delineate the track for dissection

3. Incision
   (i) Lower
       Elliptical in a skin crease around the fistula opening

(ii) Upper
     Transverse in a skin crease at the junction of the upper
     third and middle third of the neck over the anterior
     border of stermoastoid
4. Procedure
     (i) Sharply dissect out the lower fistula track *en bloc* with
         the fistula opening (this may be assisted with a probe
         lying in the track)
     (ii) Dissect the track up towards the second incision deep to
          the platysma, elevating the skin flap off the fistula track.
     (iii) Pull the specimen through to the second incision and
           continue the dissection up to the point where it *passes
           over the hypoglossal nerve*
     (iv) Continue the dissection of the track as it passes
          between:
          a. *External carotid artery* anteriorly
          b. *Internal carotid artery* posteriorly
             to join the wall of the pharynx at the posterior fauces
     (v) Ligate the fistula track and excise the specimen
5. Closure
     (i) Absolute haemastasis
     (ii) Suction drain
     (iii) Close in layers
6. Postoperative management
     (i) Remove the drain when dry (24 hours)
     (ii) Histology of fistula track
7. Complications
     (i) Uncommon
     (ii) Incomplete excision may cause recurrence of a branchial
          cyst
     (iii) Damage to *Hypoglossal nerve*

EXCISION OF PHARYNGEAL POUCH

1. Preoperative management
     (i) Investigations
         a. Barium swallow
         b. Oesophagoscopy (there is a risk of perforation of the
            pouch with careless instrumentation)
     (ii) Chest physiotherapy, since often these patients are
          elderly with a history of aspiration of pouch contents
2. Pre-incision
     (i) General anaesthesia and endotracheal intubation
     (ii) Position
          Supine
     (iii) Prior to towelling up, perform direct pharyngoscopy and
           pack the pouch either by the traditional method of a
           half-inch ribbon gauze dyed with flavine or with the
           inflated balloon of a Foley catheter

    (iv) Skin preparation of mouth to nipples and towel up to expose all of the neck
3. Incision
    (i) On the side to which the pouch is directed (90% to the left)
    (ii) Transverse across the lower third of sternomastoid on the affected side
4. Procedure
    (i) Divide the deep cervical fascia along the anterior border of sternomastoid and retract the muscle posteriorly
    (ii) Divide the tendonous mid-point of omohyoid to expose the carotid sheath
    (iii) Ligate and divide middle thyroid vein and the inferior thyroid artery if it crosses the operative field
    (iv) Gently retract
        a. Thyroid medially
        b. Carotid sheath laterally
           thus exposing the pouch
    (v) Mobilise the pouch in the neck by sharp dissection and when it is free remove the preplaced pack or balloon
    (vi) Excise the sac at its neck, flush with the pharyngeal wall between thyropharyngeus superiorly and cricopharyngeus inferiorly
    (vii) Perform a cricopharyngeus myotomy
    (viii) Close the pharyngeal defect in two layers
5. Closure
    (i) Place
        a. Fine bore soft nasogastric feeding tube
        b. Suction type drain to the wound
    (ii) Close in layers
6. Postoperative management
    (i) Remove the drains when dry at 24–48 hours
    (ii) Feed via nasogastric tube from first postoperative day
    (iii) Barium swallow at the 5th postoperative day to check the pharyngeal closure; allow to eat and drink if there is no leakage
7. Complications
    (i) Pharyngeal fistula
    (ii) Recurrent pouch (if the excision is inadequate)

BLOCK DISSECTION TO THE NECK

1. Indications
    (i) Lymph node metastases from primary head malignancies, especially
        a. Carcinoma of the lip, floor of mouth, tongue and skin
        b. Malignant melanoma

    (ii) Thyroid malignancy
       a. Papillary
       b. Medullary
   (iii) Salivary malignancy
   (iv) Lymph node recurrence after radiotherapy to cervical node metastases
    (v) Tuberculosis with the failure of chemotherapy and the absence of suppuration
2. Anatomical consideration of dissection
    (i) To remove the structure of the digastric triangle
      a. Submandibular gland
      b. Submandibular nodes
   (ii) To remove internal jugular vein (IJV)
   (iii) To remove deep cervical chain of lymph node
      a. Upper anterior sternomastoid group
      b. Upper posterior sternomastoid group
      c. Lower anterior sternomastoid group
      d. Lower posterior sternomastoid group
   (iv) To remove sternocleido mastoid node
3. Preoperative management — Determine primary pathology
    (i) Clinical examination
   (ii) Endoscopy with biopsy/brush cytology
   (iii) Radiology
      a. Primary pathology
      b. Bone involvement
      c. Contrast studies
      d. Lymphangiogram
      e. CT
   (iv) Skin test
      a. Heaf/mantoux for TB
      b. Kveim for sarcoid
    (v) Sputum
      a. Cytology
      b. Culture/AFBs
   (vi) Fine needle aspiration cytology
4. Pre-incision
    (i) General anaesthesia with endotracheal intubation
   (ii) Position
     Supine with neck extended and head turned away
   (iii) Skin preparation of mid face to lower chest, towelled up to expose all of neck
   (iv) Mark out skin incision with a marker pen
5. Incision
   Semicircular. Commence at the midline just below the mandible and descend curving outwards to a point on the lateral border sternomastoid 2 cm above the clavicle and then curve upwards to the mastoid process, including platysma with the skin

6. Procedure
    (i) Ligate and divide the external jugular vein
    (ii) Elevate the skin flap with platysma for the whole width of the incision to the top of the neck
    (iii) Divide the origin of sternomastoid 2.5 cm above the clavicle and retract upwards to expose the internal jugular vein in the carotid sheath
    (iv) Ligate and divide the internal jugular vein at the root of the neck
    (v) Gently dissect the internal jugular vein, deep cervical lymph nodes and sternomastoid *en bloc* off the carotid artery
    (vi) *Beware*
        a. *Vagus nerve* between the IJV and the carotid artery
        b. *Phrenic nerve* appearing from behind the scalenous anterior in the posterior triangle
        c. *Thoracic duct* on left
        d. *Hypoglossal nerve* crossing the external and internal carotid arteries laterally above the carotid bifurcation, and giving off the *descendens hypoglossi*
    (vii) Ligate and divide any branches of the IJV in the neck, especially the common facial vein
    (viii) Continue the dissection to the base of the skull and ligate and divide the origin of the IJV, excise the mastoid head of sternomastoid and remove the specimen en-bloc
    (ix) The dissection may continue into the anterior triangle to include the contents of the digastric triangle
7. Closure
    (i) Meticulous haemostasis
    (ii) 1 or 2 suction drains
    (iii) Apposition of platysma
    (iv) Close the skin with interrupted sutures
8. Postoperative management
    (i) Continue suction drainage for several days until the drainage is minimal
    (ii) Histological examination of the specimen
9. Complications
    (i) Early
        a. Seroma under the skin flap
        b. Skin flap necrosis, especially with incisions which involve the apposition of three or more skin flaps
        c. Raised intracranial pressure uncommon, only occurs with simultaneous bilateral block dissections
    (ii) Late
    Disease recurrence

Cardiothoracic surgery

RIGID OESOPHAGOSCOPY AND DILATATION

1. Preoperative management
   - (i) Investigations
     - a. Barium swallow
     - b. Chest X-ray
     - c. Group and save for dilatation
   - (ii) Warn patient of the possible risk of oesophageal perforation
2. Pre procedure
   - (i) General anaesthetic with endotracheal intubation, the tube placed to the left of the mouth
   - (ii) Position
     Supine with the neck supported and initially flexed. Flex the head on the neck as the scope is introduced into the mouth
   - (iii) Surgeon stands behind the patient's head, wearing protective glasses
   - (iv) Protect the patient's eyes with a towel
3. Procedure
   - (i) Select the appropriate Negus oesophagoscope (small, medium or large) according to the size of the patient
   - (ii) Pass the oesophagoscope to the back of the oropharynx extending the head on the neck in the process. Visualise the epiglottis and cords
   - (iii) Gently pass the 'scope through cricopharyngeus, extending the neck slowly as the 'scope passes down the proximal oesophagus, allowing for the thoracic kyphosis
   - (iv) As the 'scope reaches the cardia, the neck should be fully extended
   - (v) *Be very careful*
     - a. With patients with rheumatoid arthritis when extending the neck [all should have a preoperative cervical spine X-ray (see principles of surgery for rheumatoid arthritis, page 164)

      b. With patients with osteoarthritis who may have
         severe thoracic spine osteophytes (who should have
         a preoperative lateral chest X-ray)
   (vi) Visualise the pathology
      a. Biopsy/brush cytology
      b. Dilate the stricture
      c. Dilators — Chevalliere Jackson bougies
                Porges gum elastic bougie
                Maloney mercury filled bougies
  (vii) Remove the 'scope
4. Postoperative management
Chest X-ray following dilatation, the patient must remain nil
by mouth until this is seen and reported as normal by the
surgeon
5. Complications
   (i) Oesophageal perforation
  (ii) Aspiration (especially after intubation of a low
      oesophageal stricture)
 (iii) Recurrent stricture

RIGID BRONCHOSCOPY

1. Preoperative management
   (i) Chest X-rays
      a. PA and lateral
      b. Tomography of lesion
      c. (CT)
  (ii) Sputum
      a. Culture
      b. AFBs
      c. Cytology
 (iii) Skin testing
      a. Heaf test
      b. Kveim test
Preoperative physiotherapy with mucolytics and
bronchodilators in chronic obstructive airways disease (see
principles of prevention and treatment of pulmonary
problems during operations, page 10)
2. Pre procedure
   (i) General anaesthetic
  (ii) Position
      Supine with shoulders supported, neck in neutral
      position and the head flexed on the neck
 (iii) Surgeon standing behind the patient's head wearing
      protective glasses
 (iv) Towel placed to protect the patient's eyes

3. Procedure
    (i) Select a bronchoscope of appropriate size (large adult, small adult, child, infant, neonate)
    (ii) Once anaesthetic has been induced pass the 'scope over the back of the tongue and extend the head on the neck. Depress the larynx with the left hand, passing the scope behind the epiglottis under direct vision to see the vocal cords
    (iii) Gently pass the 'scope through the vocal cords into the trachea
    (iv) Negotiate down the trachea to the carina and measure its' distance from the teeth
    (v) Visualise the normal bronchial tree first by passing the 'scope down the main bronchus and using angled telescopes to look into the major segment bronchi
    (vi) Now visualise the abnormal bronchial tree, repeating the procedure
        a. Take brush cytology/biopsy specimens
        b. Remove foreign material/bodies
        c. Trap sputum — Cytology
                                  Culture
    (vii) Remove the 'scope
4. Postoperative management
    Obtain results from specimens removed
5. Complications
    Haemoptysis
    a. Rough handling
    b. Biopsy of vascular lesion

POSTEROLATERAL THORACOTOMY

1. Preoperative management
    (i) Commence physiotherapy and breathing exercises
    (ii) Examine and mark the side, shave the chest and axilla
    (iii) Investigations
        a. Chest X-ray (PA and lateral)
        b. Cross-match blood appropriate to procedure
        c. Bronchoscopy ⎫ Results relevant
        d. Oesophagoscopy ⎬ to the pathology
        e. Mediastinoscopy ⎭
    (iv) Prophylactic antibiotics, ampicillin and flucloxacillin
    (v) Intravenous infusion
    (vi) Catheter
2. Pre-incision
    (i) General anaesthetic with a double lumen endotracheal tube (eg Robertshaw)
    (ii) Position
        Lateral, with upper arm supported and the patient's back

perpendicular to the edge of the operating table, support
the upper leg with a pillow
   (iii) Skin preparation of all of back from the nape of the
neck to the small of the back and extending to the
midline at the front
   (iv) Towel up to expose the posterior and subaxillary
hemithorax
3. Incision
Commence 8 cm lateral to the 6th thoracic spinous process
and curve forward, 2 cm below the tip of the scapula to the
mid axillary line in the line of the ribs
4. Procedure
   (i) With the cutting diathermy divide:
      a. Latissimus dorsi
      b. Serratus anterior
      in the line of the incision
   (ii) Retract the lower scapula and count the ribs by
palpation from the top (the uppermost being the
second rib) as far as the 6th rib
   (iv) Elevate the periostium of the 6th rib for the length of
the incision and clear the periostium completely off the
circumference of the posterior 3 cm of the rib with
Doyen's periostial elevator
   (v) Divide the posterior end of the rib with a bone cutter
and elevate the rib from its periostial bed via its
superior edge (reducing the risk of damage to the
intercostal neurovascular bundle)
   (vi) Gently insert the rib spreader and open slowly, picking
up the parietal pleura to open it, allowing the lung to
fall away
   (vii) Open the rib spreader and divide any pleural adhesions
   (viii) Assess the pleural cavity and carry out the procedure
5. Closure
   (i) Haemostasis, swab and instrument check
   (ii) Place two pleural drains
      a. Apical for air
      b. Basal for blood
      and connect to underwater seal drainage systems
   (iii) Insert an intercostal nerve block with 0.5% Marcaine for
the intercostal space of entry and the two spaces above
and below
   (iv) Close in layers
6. Postoperative management
   (i) Chest X-ray in recovery, and then daily until the chest
drains are removed to assess lung expansion
   (ii) Nurse in a sitting position and commence postoperative
physiotherapy on the same day

(iii) Place the pleural drains on a low pressure suction pump for at least 24 hours and until the lung is fully up (5 cm water pressure on a Roberts pump)
(iv) Remove the drain when the lung is up, no air is being drained and the fluid drainage is less than 100 ml daily
(v) Methods of analgesia
  a. Marcaine intercostal block
  b. High thoracic opiate epidural
  c. Intravenous opiate infusion
7. Complications
  (i) Early
    a. Infection — Wound
                Septicaemia
                Respiratory
                Emphyema
    b. Pneumothorax
    c. Surgical emphysema
    d. Haemothorax
  (ii) Late
    a. Chronic suppuration
    b. Intercostal neuroma

MEDIAN STERNOTOMY

1. Indications
  (i) Cardiac surgery
  (ii) Surgery of the superior mediastinum (thymectomy, retrosternal thyroidectomy, surgery of the trachea and paratracheal nodes)
2. Preoperative management
  (i) Investigations
    a. Chest X-ray (PA and lateral)
    b. Cardiac investigations relevant to pathology (see principles of cardiac surgery, page 74)
    c. Bronchoscopy prior to tracheal surgery (see rigid bronchoscopy, page 67)
  (ii) Examine the legs and mark the long saphenous vein prior to coronary artery bypass graft surgery (see principles of cardiac surgery, page 74)
  (iii) Prophylactic antibiotics, ampicillin and flucloxacillin
  (iv) Intravenous line
  (v) Central venous catheter
  (vi) Arterial pressure monitor
  (vii) Bladder catheter
3. Pre-incision
  (i) General anaesthesia and endotracheal intubation
  (ii) Position
    Supine

(iii) Skin preparation of upper neck to lower abdomen, towel up to expose sternum
4. Incision
Midline from the suprasternal notch to just below the xiphoid process
5. Procedure
  (i) Divide the subcutaneous tissues to the sternal periostium with diathermy point, including the linea alba immediately below the xiphisternum
  (ii) Bluntly dissect the tissues immediately behind the xiphoid
  (iii) Divide the sternum longitudinally with a mechanical reciprocating saw
  (iv) *Beware* the pleura overlapping the mediastinum anteriorly which may be inadvertently opened
  (v) Insert a self-retaining retractor and gently open to display the pericardium inferiorly and the great vessels superiorly
  (vi) Perform appropriate surgery
6. Closure
  (i) Meticulous haemostasis
  (ii) Place two pericardial drains and bring them out below the xiphoid through separate incisions in the rectus sheath
  (iii) Pass steel wire sutures (5 metric gauge) around the sternum and twist closed to give an accurate closure
  (iv) Close the linea alba
  (v) Close the subcutaneous tissues and skin in layers
7. Postoperative management
  (i) Chest X-ray in the recovery ward — exclude *pneumothorax*
  (ii) Nurse on intensive care unit after cardiac surgery and continue ventillation at the discretion of the anaesthetist
  (iii) Remove the pericardial drains when the drainage is minimal (< 50 ml in 24 hours)
  (iv) Check the haemoglobin and transfuse accordingly
8. Complications
  (i) Early
    a. Pneumothorax
    b. Haemothorax
    c. Pericardial tamponade
    d. Those specific to cardiac surgery (see principles of cardiac surgery, page 74)
    e. Sternal dehiscence
  (ii) Late
  Keloid scar

PNEUMONECTOMY

1. Indications
   Malignant lung tumours not amenable to lobectomy
2. Preoperative management
   As for posterolateral thoracotomy, see page 68
     (i) Examine the patient, mark the side and pulmonary
        function tests
    (ii) Chest X-ray (PA and lateral)
   (iii) Tomography
    (iv) (CT)
     (v) Sputum
        a. Microbiology
        b. Cytology
    (vi) Bronchoscopy (fibreoptic/rigid)
        a. Cytology
        b. Histology
   (vii) Metastases
        Liver
        a. Function test
        b. Ultrasound
        c. Isotope scan
        Bone
        a. Skeletal survey
        b. Isotope bone scan
        Nodes
        Mediastinoscopy
3. Indications of inoperability
     (i) Evidence of metastases (including tracheal nodes)
    (ii) Tumours < 2 cm from carina
   (iii) Patient > 70 years old requiring a pneumonectomy
    (iv) Nerve involvement
        a. Recurrent laryngeal
        b. Phrenic
        c. Pancoast — T1 — Horner's syndrome
     (v) Chest wall/diaphragm invaded
    (vi) SVC obstruction
4. Relative contraindications
     (i) Blood stained pleural effusion
    (ii) Poor respiratory reserve on pulmonary function tests (FVC,
        FEV, peak flow and blood gases)
5. Pre-incision
   Perform a posterolateral thoracotomy (see page 68)
6. Procedure
     (i) Allow the lung to collapse away from the parietal
        pleura and assess the tumour (pleural, hilar and lymph
        node spread). It may be necessary to open the
        pericardium to fully assess the operability of the
        tumour

   (ii) Divide the pulmonary ligament to mobilise the lung, open the hilar pleura anteriorly
  (iii) Gently dissect out, ligate and divide the pulmonary veins
  (iv) Very carefully dissect, ligate and divide the branches of the pulmonary artery lying anterior to the main bronchus
   (v) Finally clamp and divide the bronchus, closing this with interrupted monofilament nylon or steel sutures
  (vi) Remove the specimen for histological examination
 (vii) Dissect out the subcarinal and peritracheal lymph nodes for histological examination
7. Closure
   (i) Close the pleura over the hilar stump
  (ii) Crush the phrenic nerve, allowing the diaphragm to elevate to occupy the pleural space
  (iii) No drains
  (iv) Close in layers (see posterolateral thoracotomy, page 69)
8. Postoperative management
   See posterolateral thoracotomy, page 69
   (i) Check the intra pleural pressure in the recovery room using an anaeroid manometer and two way tap, adjust to atmospheric pressure
  (ii) Nurse in a sitting position
9. Investigations
   (i) Chest X-ray
  (ii) Histology of tumour and lymph nodes
10. Complications
   (i) Early
       a. Secretion retention
       b. Surgical emphysema
       c. Pericardial cardiac herniation
       d. Empyema
       e. Broncho pleural fistula
  (ii) Late
       Tumour recurrence (75% of cases)

DRAINAGE OF EMPYEMA

1. Pathological factors
   An empyema is a pleural abscess, not just the presence of pus within the pleural cavity (pyothorax). Formal drainage should not be undertaken until an empyema is established, pyothorax should be treated by aspiration, local antibiotic instillation and systemic antibiotics
2. Preoperative management
   (i) Establish diagnosis
       a. Clinical examination

      b. Chest X-ray (PA and lateral)
      c. Needle aspiration (pus for microbiological
         examination)
   (ii) Exclude bronchopleural fistula (suggested by an air fluid
      level on the chest X-ray)
  (iii) Antibiotic cover determined by microbiological results
3. Pre-incision
    (i) Anaesthesia with local anaesthetic with mild sedation
   (ii) Position
      Sitting, with access to the back (most empyemas lie
      posteriorly)
  (iii) Skin preparation of the whole of the posterior
      hemithorax and towel up to expose a large area
      overlying the empyema
4. Incision
  Decide from the chest X-rays which rib overlies the
  empyema and incise directly over it for 8 cm
5. Procedure
    (i) Deepen in the line of the skin incision
   (ii) Infiltrate the periostium of the rib and intercostal nerve
      with local anaesthetic
  (iii) Divide the periostium and elevate this to expose the rib
  (iv) Excise 3 cm of rib and ligate the intercostal vessels at
      each end of the excision
   (v) Excise a wide disc of thickened pleura and suck out any
      free pus, sending a further specimen for microbiological
      examination
  (vi) Gently digitally break down any loculi and remove any
      solid debris with ovum forceps
 (vii) Insert a wide bore silastic chest drain and close the
      wound around it, securing the drain to the skin
(viii) Connect the drain to an underwater seal drainage
      system with low pressure suction (< 5 cm water)
6. Postoperative management
    (i) Chest X-ray in recovery ward
   (ii) After a few days cut off the drain 2–3 cm from the skin
      and leave on open, free drainage
  (iii) Daily physiotherapy
  (iv) Review collapse of the cavity with regular sinograms
7. Complications
    (i) Broncho pleural fistula from traumatic tube insertion
   (ii) Fibrous cortex to cavity — therefore, does not collapse
      and needs decortication

PRINCIPLES OF CARDIAC SURGERY

1. Preoperation
    (i) Diagnosis with

a. Echocardiography
b. Angiography
c. Electrocardiography
(ii) Treat coexisting disease
   a. Pulmonary
   b. Diabetes
   c. Peripheral vascular disease, especially carotid pathology
(iii) Check electrolytes, especially potassium (diuretics, infusion, dilution)
(iv) Anaesthetic
   a. Avoid excessive O_2 demand
   b. Decrease sympathetic activity
   c. Increase PaO_2

2. Peroperative
(i) Hypothermia
   a. systemic
   b. pericardial
(ii) Approach heart via median sternotomy (see page 70)
(iii) Cardiopulmonary bypass (extra corporeal circulation)
   a. Needs heparinisation, which is reversed at the end by protamine
   b. Gas and heat interchange
   c. Arrest heart in diastole (myocardium is at maximal relaxation)
   d. Cardioplegia — Cold
                  Potassium chloride (eg St Thomas' solution)
   e. Drain venae cavae to the pump and return blood to the aortic arch
   f. Cross clamp the aortic root (decreases the loss of cardioplegic drugs and blood)
   g. Cardiovent at the end of the procedure
   h. Remove air
(iv) During the procedure, monitor
   a. Serum potassium
   b. PaO_2 (> 10 KPa)
   c. Urine output (> 1 ml/minute)
   d. Mean arterial pressure (> 60 mmHg)

3. Post surgery — Monitor
(i) Pulse and arterial pressure
(ii) ECG
(iii) Central venous pressure
(iv) Urine output
(v) Potassium
(vi) Blood gases on ventilation

A. Valve surgery
1. Indications for surgery
   (i) Failure of medical treatment
   (ii) Regurgitation with poor compensation
2. Methods
   (i) Valvotomy
      a. Closed
      b. Open
   (ii) Plastic repair of valve
   (iii) Mechanical valve replacement
      e.g.
      a. Starr Edwards (ball and cage)
      b. Bjork Shilley (tilting disc)
      c. Advantages — Convenience
                      Easily sewn in
                      Durability
         Therefore useful for younger patients
      d. Disadvantages — Clotting and embolisation
         Therefore useful for younger patients
   (iv) Biological valve replacement
      a. Cadaveric homograft
         — Advantage   — No clotting problems
         — Disadvantages — Limited supply
                            Difficult implantation
                            'Wears out', usually within 8
                            years
      b. Porcine xenograft
         — Advantages   — Good supply
                            Glutaraldehyde treatment
                            sterilises the graft and
                            strengthens the structure
                            Easier to suture in place
                            Minimal risk of embolism
                            (therefore does not need
                            warfarin)
         — Disadvantage   — Calcify, especially in younger
                            children
3. Operative mortality
   (i) Single valve — 5–8% (8–10% if combined with coronary
       artery bypass graft)
   (ii) Multiple valve — 10–12%
4. Complications of valve replacement
   (i) Thrombosis
   (ii) Embolism
      a. Vegetation
      b. Valve — In part
                 All of valve

    (iii) Infection
       a. Early — *Staphylococcus*
       b. Late — *Streptococcus viridans*
    (iv) Paravalvular leak

B. Surgery for coronary artery disease
1. Indications
    (i) Disabling angina despite full medical treatment with proximal arterial stenosis (> 70% stenosis)
    (ii) Crescendo angina
    (iii) Post myocardial infarction
       a. Left ventricular aneurysm
       b. Ventriculo septal defect
       c. Ruptured papillary muscle
2. Preoperative investigations
    (i) Exclude life threatening peripheral vascular disease, especially carotid pathology
    (ii) Blood
       a. Lipids/cholesterol
       b. Blood sugar
       c. Plasma viscosity/packed cell volume
    (iii) ECG and stress ECG studies
    (iv) Angiography
       a. Proximal stenosis
       b. Stenosis > 70%
    (v) (Echocardiography)
    (vi) Mark out saphenous vein
3. Method
    (i) Dissect out saphenous vein, ligating all branches and marking the direction of blood flow
    (ii) Median sternotomy to expose the heart and initiate cardiopulmonary bypass with cardioplegia
    (iii) Perform vein bypasses from aorta (side-to-end anastomosis) to distal coronary artery (end-to-side anastomosis). Reversing the vein.
    (iv) Other methods
       a. Endarterectomy (proximal short stenosis)
       b. Single snake graft with multiple anastomoses
       c. Internal mammary coronary anastomosis
4. Operative mortality — 4% — Results
    (i) Asymptomatic — 70%
    (ii) Improvement in angina — 12%
    (iii) No improvement — 13%
    (iv) Early death — 4%
    (v) Late death — 3%
5. Complications
    (i) Peroperative infarction

(ii) Stroke
   a. Unsuspected carotid stenosis
   b. Embolism
(iii) Late graft occlusion

REPAIR OF AORTIC COARCTATION

1. Indications for surgery
   (i) Infancy
      a. Left ventricular failure
      b. In combination with surgery for other anomalies
   (ii) Children
      Before 6 years old and onset of hypertension
2. Preoperative management
   (i) Correct congestive cardiac failure and hypertension as much as is possible (although in an emergency this must not postpone surgery)
   (ii) Investigations
      a. Aortography   — Delineate coarctation
         Pressure gradient studies
         Exclude patent ductus arteriosus
      b. Echocardiography — Exclude coexistent aortic and mitral valve abnormalities
         ECG — Left ventricular hypertrophy
         CXR — May show rib notching in older children
   (iii) Broad spectrum antibiotic prophylaxis
   (iv) Continuous monitor
      a. IVI
      b. CVP
      c. Pulmonary wedge pressure
      d. Arterial pressure
      e. ECG
      f. Catheterise bladder
3. Pre-incision
   (i) General anaesthesia with double lumen endotracheal tube to allow collapse of left lung. Careful peroperative control of blood pressure with sodium nitro-prusside
   (ii) Perform an extended left posterolateral thoracotomy (see page 68)
   (iii) Beware distended chest wall collateral vessels
4. Procedure
   (i) Divide the mediastinal pleura vertically from the left subclavian artery to well below the coarctation
   (ii) *Beware the vagus nerve overlying aortic arch*
   (iii) Ligate and divide the left superior intercostal vein

(iv) Mobilise the left subclavian artery, distal aortic arch, coarctation and descending aorta and place slings around these vessels
(v) Ligate and divide the ligamentum/ductus arteriosum
(vi) *Beware the left recurrent laryngeal nerve arching under aorta*
(vii) Place clamps to control the aorta above and below the coarctation
(viii) Excise the coarctation and perform an end-to-end anastomosis to repair the aorta
(ix) Problems
   a. Long coarctation — Dacron patch aortoplasty
                           Dacron tube graft
   b. Infantile preductal coarctation — Subclavian flap operation
   c. Inadequate collateral circulation impairs peroperative renal perfusion (pressure in descending aorta < < 50 mmHg) — Use left atriofemoral bypass
5. Closure
   (i) Repair the parietal pleura
   (ii) Close as posterolateral thoracotomy (page 69)
6. Postoperative management
   (i) Monitor in an intensive care unit until stable
   (ii) Monitor cardiac function
      a. Arterial pressure
      b. CVP
      c. Pulmonary wedge pressure
      d. ECG
   (iii) Monitor renal function
      a. Output
      b. Electrolytes
      c. Osmolality
7. Operative mortality
   (i) Infant with other anomalies > 10%
   (ii) Childhood — 2%
   (iii) Adult — 2–5%
8. Complications
   (i) Early
      a. Haemorrhage (especially chest wall collaterals)
      b. Recurrent laryngeal nerve palsy
      c. Chylothorax
      d. Paraplegia
      e. Acute renal failure
   (ii) Late
      a. Persistent hypertension (if longstanding coarctation resulted in renal changes)
      b. Recurrent coarctation

CLOSURE OF PATENT DUCTUS ARTERIOSUS

1. Indications for surgery
    (i) Left ventricular failure
    (ii) Aneurysmal dilatation of the ductus
    (iii) Bacterial endocarditis
2. Contra-indications for surgery
    Severe pulmonary hypertension with shunt reversal
3. Preoperative management
    (i) Cardiac catheterisation
        a. Confirm diagnosis
        b. Exclude coexistent abnormalities
        c. Measure pulmonary vascular resistence
    (ii) Timing of surgery
        a. Ideally between age 2–5 years
        b. Onset of complications
    (iii) Broad spectrum antibiotic prophylaxis
    (iv) IVI
    (v) Catheterise
    (vi) Systemic and pulmonary arterial pressure monitor
    (vii) ECG monitor
4. Pre-incision
    (i) General anaesthesia with double lumen endotracheal
        intubation to allow deflation of the left lung
    (ii) Perform left lateral thoracotomy (see page 68)
5. Procedure
    (i) Allow the lung to collapse and retract it forwards
    (ii) Incise the mediastinal pleura overlying the aorta from
        proximal to the origin of the left subclavian artery to
        below the ductus which can be palpated as a thrill
    (iii) Gently mobilise the aorta and place tapes proximally
        and distally
    (iv) Retraction on the tapes displays the ductus, left vagus
        and left recurrent laryngeal nerve passing under the
        ductus
    (v) Test clamp the ductus
        If there is no fall in pulmonary artery pressure then
        abandon the operation
    (vi) Doubly ligate the ductus with a non-absorbable suture
6. Closure
    Close the parietal pleura (see posterolateral thoracotomy,
    page 69)
7. Postoperative management
    (i) Nurse on an intensive care unit until stable
    (ii) Investigate pulmonary artery pressures
8. Complications
    Operative mortality
    a. Children without pulmonary hypertension — 0.5%

b. Children with pulmonary hypertension and adults — 1.0%
Ductus recanalisation < 0.1%

PRINCIPLES OF OESOPHAGECTOMY

1. Indications
    (i) Adenocarcinoma of the cardia or arising within ectopic gastric mucosa (Barratt's oesophagus)
    (ii) Squamous carcinoma of the oesophagus (results are comparable with radiotherapy)
    (iii) Benign oesophageal stricture not amenable to dilatation and antireflux procedures
2. Pathological factors
    (i) 90% of malignancy is squamous carcinoma
    (ii) 10% of malignancy is adenocarcinoma
    (iii) Direct spread is early since the oesophagus has no serosa and submucosal spread is extensive
    (iv) Lymphatic spread is early
    (v) Sites of tumours
        a. Upper third — 15%
        b. Middle third — 50%
        c. Lower third — 35%
    (vi) Because of dysphagia these patients are often in a poor state of nutrition at presentation
3. Preoperative management
    (i) Investigations
        a. Barium swallow
        b. Chest X-ray
        c. Oesophagoscopy and biopsy (see page 66)
        d. Bronchoscopy for tumours of upper and mid third (see page 67)
        e. Metastases — Liver — Liver function tests
                                      Ultrasound
                                      Isotope liver scan
    (ii) If malnourished, then correct the catabolic effect for at least 10 days prior to surgery
        a. Enterally — Nasogastric tube
                             Gastrostomy
        b. Parenterally
    (iii) Chest physiotherapy
    (iv) Bowel preparation (see page 116) if colonic interposition anticipated
    (v) Antibiotic prophylaxis; broad spectrum (metronidazole if colonic interposition anticipated)
    (vi) IVI
    (vii) Catheter
    (viii) CVP monitor

A. **Tumour at 35–40 cm from the teeth**
    (i) Use a left thoracoabdominal incision
    (ii) The limit to this approach is the arch of the aorta which crosses the mid third of the oesophagus
    (iii) Position left semi lateral

1. Incision
Oblique commencing to the right of the midline in the epigastrium and up to the left costal margin and extended via the bed of the left 7th rib posteriorly to the posterior axillary line

2. Procedure
    (i) Full laparotomy, exclude liver and peritoneal metastases
    (ii) Divide the diaphragm circumferentially to protect the innervation of the phrenic nerve
    (iii) Mobilise the stomach by dividing the left gastric vessels, short gastric vessels and left gastroepiploic vessels
    (iv) Divide the left pulmonary ligament to improve access to the oesophagus
    (v) Mobilise the lower third of the oesophagus
    (vi) Resect the specimen
    (vii) Reconstruction for squamous carcinoma of the lower third
       a. Resect only the upper half of the stomach and anastomose the distal gastric remnant to the lower oesophagus
       b. If the gap is too great then manage as (viii)
    (viii) Reconstruction for adenocarcinoma
       a. Perform total gastrectomy (to reduce the 'cancer field')
       b. Create anastomosis with proximal jejunum as Roux-en-Y loop to the oesophagus

3. Closure
    (i) Drain the anastomoses and the left pleural space
    (ii) Close in layers

B. **Tumour at 25–35 cm from the teeth**
    (i) Use the Ivor Lewis method
    (ii) Position, initially, supine
    (iii) Perform an upper midline incision and a full laparotomy (exclude liver and peritoneal metastases)
    (iv) Mobilise the upper stomach (divide left gastric, short gastric and left gastroepiploic vessels)
    (v) Close the abdominal incision
    (vi) Place in right lateral position
    (vii) Perform a right posterolateral thoracotomy (see page 68)

(viii) Divide the right pulmonary ligament and the agygos vein as it crosses the oesophagus
(ix) Gently mobilise the oesophagus and tumour and pull through the proximal stomach into the chest
(x) Resect the tumour
(xi) Anastomose the proximal stomach to the upper oesophagus

Closure
(i) Drain the anastomosis and the right pleural space
(ii) Close in layers (see posterolateral thoracotomy, see page 69)

C. Tumour at 15–25 cm from the teeth
1. Good case to treat by radiotherapy alone (5000 rads in fractions over 4–5 weeks)
2. Operation
   (i) Use the McKeown method
   (ii) First two stages as for the Ivor Lewis method without resection within the chest
3. The third stage of the procedure is a right cervical incision and mobilisation of the cervical oesophagus from which the oesophageal specimen is withdrawn, delivering the proximal stomach to the neck
4. Resect the tumour and anastomose the proximal stomach to the hypopharynx
5. Closure
   (i) Drain
      a. Cervical anastomosis
      b. Right pleural space
   (ii) Close in layers
6. Alternative method
   (i) Replace the oesophagus with mobilised transverse colon based on a pedicle of left upper colic artery supported by the mariginal artery, lying either in the oesophageal bed, retrosternally or subcutaneously presternally, this needs
      a. Preoperative bowel preparation (see page 116)
      b. Antibiotic prophylaxis for gram negative organisms and anaerobes
      c. A further anastomosis, mobilising the right hemicolon and anastomosing it to the left hemicolon

Postoperative management
1. Investigations
   (i) Chest X-ray in recovery: exclude a pneumothorax in the opposite hemithorax to that which has been operated on
   (ii) Histology of specimen

    (iii) Barium swallow at 5 days post surgery —
         Anastomosis — Patency
                        Leaks
                        Gastric emptying, since
                        truncal vagotomy is
                        inevitable with
                        oesophagectomy
2. Remove drains when swallowing normally with no leaks from anastomosis
3. Consider parenteral nutrition in postoperative phase
4. Complications
    (i) Early
       a. Respiratory problems common (see page 10)
       b. Anastomotic leakage and fistulae
       c. Pneumothorax
    (ii) Late
       a. Anastomotic stricture — Fibrous
                                       Tumour recurrence
       b. Distant tumour recurrence
    (iii) Mortality
       a. Operative — 10–20%
       b. 5-year survival < 15%
    (iv) Inoperable tumour
       a. Locally fixed squamous carcinoma then treat with radiotherapy
       b. Metastatic squamous carcinoma or adenocarcinoma — Consider palliative intubation to relieve dysphagia
       Endoscopically placed tube
       a. Atkinson's modification of Celestin tube
       b. Souttars tube
       Surgically placed tube
       a. Celestin's tube
       b. Mousseau-Barbin's tube
         (Many other tubes are commercially available)

Upper gastrointestinal surgery

HELLERS OPERATION FOR ACHALASIA

1. Indications for surgery
   (i) Failure of conservative treatment (hydrostatic bag)
   (ii) Worsening achalasia
   (iii) Secondary organic changes within the oesophagus (ulceration)
   (iv) Pulmonary complications
2. Preoperative management
   (i) Investigations
      a. Barium swallow
      b. Oesophagoscopy and biopsy to exclude malignant stricture
      c. Oesophageal manometry
   (ii) Correct nutritional status, since these patients are often malnourished at the time of presentation
   (iii) Aspirate the oesophagus and chest physiotherapy as there is a significant risk of aspiration of oesophageal contents
   (iv) IVI
   (v) Nasogastric tube
3. Pre-incision
   (i) General anaesthesia with endotracheal intubation
   (ii) Position
      Supine
   (iii) Skin preparation for an upper abdominal incision
4. Incision
   Upper midline
5. Procedure
   (i) Full laparotomy, examine the cardia to exclude any other causes of dysphagia
   (ii) Retract the left lobe of the liver medially to expose the abdominal oesophagus
   (iii) Divide the peritoneum overlying the oesophagus and gently mobilise the oesophagus. Place a sling around the oesophagus

(iv) Divide the transverse vessels at the cardia between ligatures

(v) Commence the myotomy immediately below the cardia on the stomach and extend it upwards longitudinally on the anterior oesophagus to the point where it is clearly dilated

(vi) *Beware anterior vagus nerve* — Lying on oesophagus
   a. Damage during oesophageal traction to —
      Left gastric vessels
      Short gastric vessel
      Spleen
   b. Perforating the mucosa during seromyotomy (close with absorbable suture)

(vii) Suture the fundus of the stomach to the left and then the right edges of the myotomy folding the fundus across anteriorly (Dor procedure)

(viii) Closure
   a. Haemostasis
   b. No drains
   c. Close abdomen in layers

6. Postoperative management
   (i) Remove the nasogastric tube and commence oral fluids the next day
   (ii) Investigations only if symptoms persist, then repeat investigations for achalasia
   (iii) Complications (early)
      a. Peritonitis with missed mucosal perforation
      b. Persistent dysphagia — Either oedema from manipulation at surgery or incomplete myotomy
      c. Reactionary haemorrhage from spleen or short gastric vessels

SURGERY FOR GASTRO OESOPHAGEAL REFLUX AND HIATUS HERNIA

1. Aim of surgery
   To restore and maintain an intra-abdominal segment of oesophagus

2. Indications for surgery
   (i) Gastro oesophageal reflux
      a. Failure of medical treatment for intractible symptoms
      b. Complications — Peptic ulcer
                        Peptic stricture
                        Carcinoma
                        Haemorrhage
                        Recurrent aspiration

(ii) Sliding hiatus hernia if associated with indications to operate for gastro oesophageal reflux

(iii) Rolling hiatus hernia almost always should be operated because of the risk of strangulation of either the fundus or small bowel within the sac and the associated risk risk of gastric volvulus

3. Principles of surgery
    (i) Restore intra-abdominal oesophagus
    (ii) Create an oesophageal 'valve' or 'flap'
    (iii) Perform repair of hiatus around a soft oesophageal bougie or tube, so it is not too tight
    (iv) Preserve vagi
    (v) Investigations
        a. Chest X-ray
        b. Barium swallow
        c. Oesophagoscopy and biopsy of abnormal tissue to exclude malignancy
        d. Intra-oesophageal pH monitor
        e. Bernstein test (acid perfusion of lower oesophagus to reproduce the symptoms of oesophagitis)
        f. Oesophageal manometry

BELSEY MARK IV ANTI-REFLUX OPERATION

1. Pre-incision
    (i) General anaesthetic with a double lumen endotracheal tube to allow deflation of the left lung
    (ii) Position
        Right lateral
    (iii) Skin preparation for left posterolateral thoracotomy
2. Incision
    Left posterolateral thoracotomy via the bed of the 7th rib (see page 68)
3. Procedure
    (i) Allow lung to deflate and divide the left pulmonary ligament
    (ii) Divide the pleura overlying the oesophagus below the aortic arch and mobilise the oesophagus. Place a sling around it
    (iii) Ligate and divide the oesophageal branches of the aorta
    (iv) *Beware*
        a. Opening the opposite pleural space
        b. Damage to the vagi
    (v) Open the peritoneal sac lying anterior to the thoracic stomach and divide the phreno-oesophageal ligament
    (vi) The stomach and oesophagus are now completely free within the chest

(vii) Perform the fundoplication in two rows of interrupted
sutures around the anterolateral three-quarters of the
oesophagus (leaving the posterior quarter of the
oesophageal circumference bare)
   a. The first row of sutures buttress the fundus to the
oesophagus
   b. The second row of sutures buttress the fundus and
oesophagus to the diaphragm
(viii) Close any residual hiatal deficit with interrupted sutures
after the fundoplication has reduced the stomach and
lower oesophagus to the abdomen
(ix) Closure
   a. Drain the hemithorax via an underwater seal drain
   b. Reinflate the left lung and close the thoracotomy
    (see page 69)
4. Postoperative management
  (i) Chest X-ray in recovery
   a. Ensure left lung is fully inflated
   b. Exclude right pneumothorax
  (ii) Commence nasogastric tube feeding on the first
postoperaive day
  (iii) Remove
   a. Chest drain when the drainage is minimal (2–3 days)
   b. Nasogastric tube at 2–3 days, then continue free
fluids until the 6th postoperative day when solids can
commence
5. Complications
  (i) Early
   a. Right side pneumothorax
   b. Early dysphagia is very common and usually resolves
  (ii) Late
   a. Recurrent gastro-oesophageal reflux (10%)
   b. Stricture at cardia

NISSEN FUNDOPLICATION

1. Pre-incision
  (i) General anaesthesia with endotracheal intubation
  (ii) Position
    Supine
  (iii) Skin preparation for an upper abdominal incision
2. Incision
  Upper midline
3. Procedure
  (i) Full laparotomy
  (ii) Retract the left lobe of the liver medially
  (iii) Mobilise the gastric fundus by
   a. Ligating and dividing the short gastric vessels

b. Ligating and dividing the upper branches of the left
   gastric artery
c. Divide the peritoneum overlying the oesophagus
(iv) *Beware* damage to the spleen
(v) Reduce the hiatus hernia if present
(vi) Draw the fundus around the posterior oesophagus and
   perform the fundoplication by suturing its apex loosely
   to the anterior lower oesophagus and upper body of the
   stomach with several interrupted non-absorbable sutures
(vii) Repair any hiatal deficit with several non-absorbable
   mattress sutures
4. Closure
   (i) No drains
   (ii) Close in layers
5. Postoperative management
   Remove the nasogastric tube on the first postoperative day
   and commence oral fluids
6. Complications
   (i) Early
      a. Acute gastric dilatation
      b. Reactionary haemorrhage
      c. Gastric fistula
      d. Dysphagia (usually transient)
   (ii) Late
      Recurrent gastro-oesophageal reflux

ANGELCHIK PROSTHESIS OPERATION

(i) Proceed as for a Nissen fundoplication as far as
   retraction of the left lobe of the liver (see page 88)
(ii) Divide the peritoneum lying anteriorly over the lower
   oesophagus and continue laterally around both sides of
   the oesophagus until the lowest 2–3 cm of oesophagus
   is fully mobilised
(iii) Gently insert the silicone prosthesis around the lower
   oesophagus and tie the two ties at the free ends
   together
(iv) Repair any hiatal deficit with several non-absorbable
   mattress sutures

Closure and postoperative management
As for Nissen fundoplication (see above)

PRINCIPLES OF PEPTIC ULCER SURGERY

1. Establish the diagnosis
   Investigations
   a. Endoscopy with biopsy

b. Barium meal
c. Gastric function tests — Resting (basal) acid secretion
                              Pentagastrin stimulation test
d. Hormone assay — Gastrin (Zollinger-Ellison) — Calcium
                                                  challenge
                                                  Secretin
                                                  challenge

Note: DU = duodenal ulcer; PPU = prepyloric ulcer; GU = gastric ulcer

Operation for benign gastric ulcer (including prepyloric ulcers)

	Recurrence (%)	Mortality (%)
Billroth I gastrectomy (including ulcer site)	7	2
Truncal vagotomy, pyloroplasty and excision of ulcer	10	1
Proximal gastric vagotomy and excision of ulcer	10 — GU 30 — PPU	1
Vagotomy and antrectomy (for prepyloric ulcer)	2	2

Operation for duodenal ulcer (including prepyloric ulcers)

	Recurrence (%)	Mortality (%)
Gastrojejunostomy	40 (including stomal)	1
Billroth II gastrectomy	10 (stomal)	2
Truncal vagotomy and drainage (pyloroplasty, gastroenterostomy)	5–15	1
Proximal gastric vagotomy	5–15	0.05
Truncal vagotomy and antrectomy	2	2

2. Reasons for recurrent GU
   (i) Persistence of aetiological factors
       a. Non steroidal anti-inflammatory drugs
       b. Steroids
   (ii) Misdiagnosed gastric carcinoma
   (iii) Delayed gastric emptying
   (iv) Inadequate gastric resection
   (v) Duodenogastric reflux

3. Reasons for recurrent DU stomal ulcer
    (i) Inadequate vagotomy
    (ii) Inadequate gastric resection (with retained antrum
         following Billroth II)
    (iii) Zollinger-Ellison syndrome
        a. G-cell hyperplasia
        b. Pancreatic gastrinoma
    (v) Hyperparathyroidism

A. **Emergency peptic ulcer surgery**
1. Bleeding PU
    (i) Conservative management
        a. Antacids   ⎱ Alone, no effect but
        b. H$_2$ antagonist ⎰ helpful in combination
    (ii) Endoscopic sclerotherapy
        a. Diathermy cautery
        b. YAG laser
2. GU
    Surgery — Billroth I or II gastrectomy including ulcer site
3. DU
    Surgery — Duodenotomy with oversew of bleeding ulcer in
    combination with definitive procedure for the ulcer (truncal
    vagotomy and pyloroplasty)
4. Perforated PU (see oversew of a perforated duodenal ulcers,
    page 94)
    (i) GU
        a. Small ulcer — Excise the ulcer (to exclude carcinoma
                         of the stomach) and close defect
        b. Large ulcer — Partial gastrectomy
    (ii) DU
        a. Early presentation — (Within 6 hours of perforation)
                                truncal vagotomy and
                                pyloroplasty which includes the
                                perforation
        b. Late presentation — (Later than 6 hours after
                                perforation or significant
                                peritoneal soiling)
                                Oversew of perforation using an
                                omental patch
    (iii) In all cases full saline peritoneal lavage and a therapeutic
         course of antibiotics (broad spectrum and metronidazole)
         commencing before the operation

TRUNCAL VAGOTOMY AND PYLOROPLASTY

1. Preoperative management
    (i) Investigations — See principles of peptic ulcer surgery,
        page 89

    (ii) Antibiotics — Cephalosporin and metronidazole as the stomach is to be opened. H_2 antagonists result in gastric bacterial colonisation and should be stopped for 48 hours prior to surgery)

    (iii) Nasogastric tube

    (iv) IVI

2. Pre-incision
   (i) General anaesthetic with endotracheal intubation
   (ii) Position Supine
   (iii) Skin preparation for an upper abdominal incision

3. Incision
   Upper midline

4. Procedure
   (i) Full laparotomy (exclude common conditions which mimic peptic ulcer symptoms: gallstones, hiatus hernia)
   (ii) Retract the left lobe of the liver medially to visualise the oesophagus at the hiatus
   (iii) Divide the peritoneum overlying the front of the oesophagus and encircle the abdominal oesophagus with an index finger, dividing the posterior peritoneal oesophageal attachment. Place a sling around the oesophagus
   (iv) *Identify, ligate and resect 1–2 cm of*
       a. *Posterior vagal trunk* — Lies up to 1 cm distant from posterior right oesophagus in the lesser omentum
           Can always be found in the angle of the hiatus
       b. *Anterior vagal trunk* — Lying on the anterior oesophagus
   (v) Send these specimens for confirmatory histological examination
   (vi) *Perform a Heinecke-Mikulicz pyloroplasty*
       a. Make a longitudinal incision extending equidistant, either side of the pylorus
       b. Close this incision transversely in two layers with interrupted sutures
       c. Closure — Haemostasis (especially the spleen)
           No drains
           Close in layers

5. Postoperative management
   (i) Regular nasogastric aspiration for 24–48 hours until the aspirate is minimal and then commence oral fluids
   (ii) Investigation
       a. Histological examination of vagal fibres
       b. Hollander insulin test or sham feeding test to confirm complete vagotomy

6. Complications
   (i) Early
      a. Leak from pyloroplasty
      b. Acute gastric dilatation (with oedematous
         pyloroplasty)
      c. Gastric atony
   (ii) Mid — failure of gastric emptying (atony)
   (iii) Late
      a. Diarrhoea
      b. Dumping
      c. Recurrent ulcer

PROXIMAL GASTRIC VAGOTOMY

Proceed as for truncal vagotomy as far as the laparotomy (see page 92)
1. Procedure
   (i) Retract the left lobe of the liver medially to expose anterior aspect of the stomach
   (ii) Identify the 'crows foot' of vessels descending onto the pylorus from the lesser omentum. Commence at the most proximal of these vessels, some 8 cm proximal to the pylorus
   (iii) Incise the peritoneum of the lesser omentum and continue this incision proximally up the lesser curve, 1 cm from the junction of lesser omentum and stomach, ligating and dividing all vessels as far as the left gastric vessels
   (iv) Return to the starting point and now ligate and divide all the small vessels lying between the two leaves of the lesser omentum for the length of the incision
   (v) Now divide the posterior leaf of the lesser omentum, ligating its vessels for the length of this incision
   (vi) Continue the incision at the proximal end of the anterior lesser omentum obliquely upwards to the angle of His, between the fundus and oesophagus, and pass a sling around the oesophagus to retract it
   (vii) Complete the division of the peritoneum from around the cardia and meticulously divide all the longitudinal nerve fibres descending around the oesophagus onto the stomach
2. Closure
   (i) Bury the bare area of stomach along the lesser curve by closing the gastric serosa over the two layers of lesser omental peritoneum with a continuous suture to reduce the risks of gastric perforation due to ischaemia
   (ii) No drain
   (iii) Close in layers

3. Postoperative management
   Commence oral fluids the next day
4. Complications
   (i) Early — Acute lesser curve necrosis
   (ii) Late — Recurrent ulcer 5–10%

OVERSEW OF A PERFORATED DUODENAL ULCER

(i) Establish the diagnosis
   a. Clinically
   b. Free gas on abdominal X-rays (80%)
   c. Leucocytosis
   d. Raised amylase (300–1000 units)
(ii) Resuscitation
   a. IVI — Restore blood pressure with colloid and, if
      anaemic, transfuse peroperatively
   b. Catheterise to monitor urine output
(iii) Antibiotics
   a. Broad spectrum and metronidazole for a full
      therapeutic course commencing at the suspicion of
      the diagnosis
   b. Analgesia for peritonitis
(iv) Uncertain diagnosis — Exclude
   a. Myocardial infarction
   b. Leaking aorta aneurysm
   c. Acute pancreatitis
   d. Acute cholecystitis
1. Pre-incision
   (i) General anaesthetic with endotracheal intubation
   (ii) Position
      Supine
   (iii) Skin preparation of the whole of the abdomen but with
      the towels placed for an upper abdominal incision
2. Incision
   Upper midline
3. Procedure
   (i) On entering the peritoneum, there is a rush of free gas,
      swab the intra-peritoneal fluid for microbiological
      examination and suck out this fluid, wipe out any large
      deposits of food or debris
   (ii) Identify the perforation and excise the free edge of the
      ulcer
   (iii) If the ulcer is small, then close transversely with
      interrupted absorbable sutures. Cover the repir with free
      greater omentum and suture in place with non-
      absorbable sutures

(iv) If the ulcer is large, then closing the defect may result in pyloric stenosis, so plug with free greater omentum and suture in place with non-absorbable sutures

(v) Full peritoneal lavage with warm saline

4. Controversies
    (i) Use of an antiseptic (e.g. *noxytyalin*) or an antibiotic (e.g. *tetracycline*) in saline lavage
    (ii) Drainage of the closure, or potential abscess (subphrenic spaces, subhepatic spaces, pelvis)

5. Closure
    (i) Haemostasis
    (ii) Swabs and instruments
    (iii) Close in layers

6. Postoperative management
    (i) Commence antacid therapy (H_2 antagonists) immediately postsurgery as no definitive surgery has been undertaken for the ulcer
    (ii) Continue nasogastric aspiration until minimal
    (iii) Commence oral fluids when bowel sounds return, nasogastric aspirate is minimal and flatus is passed per rectum

7. Complications
    (i) Early
        a. Bleeding — From ulcer edge
                      From coexistent posterior ulcer
        b. Pyloric stenosis with oedema
        c. Ileus
        d. Peritonitis
        e. Abscess — Subphrenic
                     Subhepatic
                     Pelvic
    (ii) Late
        a. Recurrent ulceration (70% if no definitive ulcer procedure has been undertaken)
        b. Obstruction from post-peritonitis adhesions

GASTRECTOMY (BILLROTH I, BILLROTH II, TOTAL)

1. Indications
    (i) Benign gastric ulcer
        a. Chronic, not responding to medical treatment
        b. Complicated — Bleeding
                         Perforated
                         Pyloric stenosis
    (ii) Carcinoma of the stomach

2. Preoperative management
   (i) Investigations
      a. Elective surgery — Haemoglobin and correct
                            anaemia if present
                            Endoscopy and biopsy
                            Barium meal
                            Benign ulcer — Gastric secretion
                            test
                            Malignant ulcer, exclude
                            metastases — Liver function tests
                                              Liver ultrasound
                                            Liver isotope scan
      b. Emergency surgery — Bleeding ulcer — Endoscopy
                                                  Transfuse
                                                Monitor CVP
                                            Perforation
                            — Plain
                              X-rays
                          — Amylase
   (ii) Tubes
      a. IVI
      b. Nasogastric tube
      c. Catheter
      d. CVP line for emergency surgery
   (iii) Antibiotics
      Broad spectrum with metronidazole
3. Pre-incision
   (i) General anaesthesia with endotracheal intubation
   (ii) Position
      Supine
   (iii) Skin preparation
      Prepare and towel up for an upper abdominal incision
4. Incision
   (i) Upper midline
   (ii) Alternatives
      a. Upper transverse
      b. Left upper paramedian
      c. Thoracoabdominal for total gastrectomy

A Billroth I gastrectomy

1. Indications
   (i) Benign gastric ulcer
   (ii) Small prepyloric carcinoma
   (iii) Acquired pyloric stenosis
2. Procedure
   (i) Full laparotomy

(ii) Open the gastrocolic omentum, divide and ligate the right gastroepiploic vessels and the distal gastric branches of the left gastroepiploic vessels
(iii) Ligate and divide the right gastric vessels
(iv) Divide the lesser omentum, ligate and divide the lower branches of the left gastric artery and vein
(v) Kocherise the duodenum and mobilise the first part of the duodenum
(vi) Place a soft bowel clamp across the first part of the duodenum and a crushing clamp across the pylorus
(vii) Place a soft clamp across the width of the mid body of the stomach, including any pathology with the distal specimen. Place a crushing clamp parallel and distal to this and excise the distal stomach within the crushing clamps
(viii) Close the gastric remnant in two layers from the lesser curve for about two-thirds of the width of the stomach
(ix) Anastomose the gastric orifice to the first part of the duodenum in two layers

B   Billroth II (Polya) gastrectomy
1. Indications
   As for Billroth I
2. Procedure
   (i) Perform gastectomy as for Billroth I as far as the removal of the specimen
   (ii) Close the duodenal stump in two layers
   (iii) Locate the duodeno-jejunal flexure and bring up the most available proximal loop of jejunum. Place a soft clamp transversely to isolate the anti-mesenteric border of 10 cm of jejunum
   (iv) Close the gastric remnant in two layers from the lesser curve for about half of the width of the stomach
   (v) Anastomose the gastric remnant in two layers to the anti-mesenteric border of the jejunal loop
       (Arguments for retrocolic versus antecolic gastrojejunostomy are probably spurious)

C   Total Gastrectomy
1. Indications
   Malignant gastric tumour
2. Procedure
   (i) Proceed as for Billroth I gastrectomy, divide the right and left gastrocolic vessels and the right gastric vessels

  (ii) Divide the left gastric vessels
 (iii) Dividing the short gastric vessels individually
 (iv) *Beware*
      a. *Spleen*
      b. *Tail of pancreas*
  (v) Place soft bowel clamps across the first part of the
      duodenum and oesophagus with crushing clamps on
      the adjacent stomach. Excise and remove the gastric
      specimen
 (vi) Close the duodenal stump in two layers
(vii) Fashion a Roux loop of 60 cm from proximal jejunum
      and anastomose this to the distal oesophagus
(viii) Closure
      a. Drain all anastomoses and duodenal stump
      b. Place a nasogastric tube
      c. Close in layers
3. Postoperative management
  (i) Investigations
      a. Check haemoglobin and transfuse accordingly
      b. Histology of specimen
 (ii) Remove
      a. Nasogastric tube when the aspirate is minimal
      b. Drains when drainage is minimal but leave the
         duodenal stump drain for 5 days (thus reducing the
         morbidity of a duodenal fistula)
(iii) Commence oral fluids with the passage of flatus per
      rectum
4. Complications
  (i) Early
      a. Gastric outflow obstruction at anastomosis — Oedema
                                                       Stricture
      b. Duodenal stump leakage with Billroth II
 (ii) Late
      a. Dumping — 90% early dumping
                   10% late dumping
      b. Nutritional — Iron deficiency
                       B_{12} deficiency
                       Calcium deficiency
      c. Weight loss
      d. Increased incidence of reactivation of tuberculosis
      e. Bilious vomiting with Billroth II gastrectomy
      f. Diarrhoea
      g. Increased incidence of gallstones
      h. Increased incidence of carcinoma of the stomach

RAMSTEDTS OPERATION FOR PYLORIC STENOSIS

1. Preoperative management
   (i) Establish the diagnosis
       a. Clinical examination
       b. Test feed
       c. Barium meal
   (ii) Correct
       a. Dehydration
       b. Metabolic alkalosis
       c. *Hypokalaemia*
   (iii) Gastric lavage via a nasogastric tube
   (iv) Nasogastric tube
   (v) IVI
2. Pre-incision
   (i) Operating theatre temperature > 17°C to reduce chilling
   (ii) General anaesthesia with endotracheal intubation
   (iii) Position
        Supine and otherwise well wrapped
   (iv) Skin preparation for an upper abdominal incision
3. Incision
   Upper right transverse (over the palpable pyloric tumour)
   muscle splitting
4. Procedure
   (i) Deliver the pyloric tumour into the incision
   (ii) Pyloromyotomy — incise the peritoneum over the length
        of the tumour and split both the longitudinal and
        circular muscle fibres down to the submucosa
   (iii) Beware
        a. Opening the duodenal mucosa, suspected if any
           bubbles of gastric juice and air appear within the
           incision
        b. If so, repair with a fine absorbable suture
5. Closure
   (i) No drains
   (ii) Close in layers
6. Postoperative management
   (i) Test feed the baby on small amounts of milk 4 hours
       after waking up and gradually increase over 48 hours
   (ii) Persistent vomiting; stop the feeds and recommence
        slowly 8 hours later
7. Complications
   (i) Early
       a. Peritonitis due to unrecognised mucosal perforation
       b. Inadequate pyloromyotomy with persistent vomiting
   (ii) Late
        Recurrent pyloric stenosis is rare

LAPAROTOMY FOR BOWEL OBSTRUCTION

1. Preoperative management
   (i) Resuscitate
       Rehydrate and correct electrolyte losses (sodium and potassium)
   (ii) Investigations
       a. Electrolytes
       b. Full blood count/PCV to assess dehydration —
          ? Anaemia
          ? leucocytosis with strangulation
       c. ECG — Effects of electrolyte disturbances
       d. AXR — Level of obstruction
          Fluid levels on erect film
          Free gas with concomittant perforation
       e. Small bowel enema/follow through
       f. NG tube — Empty the stomach prior to anaesthesia
       g. IVI
       h. Catheterise
   (iii) Broad spectrum and metronidazole antibiotic prophylaxis
2. Indications for surgery
   (i) Simple obstruction not relieved by conservative measures after 24–48 hours
   (ii) Evidence of
       a. Peritonism (pyrexia)
       b. Strangulated bowel (leucocytosis)
   (iii) Free gas on plain X-rays
3. Pre-incision
   (i) General anaesthesia and endotracheal intubation
   (ii) Position
       Supine
   (iii) Skin preparation of all of abdomen, nipples to thighs
4. Incision
   Right paramedian at the level of the umbilicus
5. Procedure
   (i) Open the peritoneum carefully: beware underlying distended bowel
   (ii) Suck out free fluid, sending a specimen for microbiological examination
6. Small bowel obstruction
   (i) Commence in right iliac fossa, looking for collapsed distal ileum
   (iii) Trace the bowel proximally from this as far as the agent of of obstruction (adhesions, intra-abdominal hernia, tumour)
   (iv) Relieve obstruction

   (v) If bowel is strangulated then increase the patient's
oxygenation, wrap in warm saline soaked packs and
review after 10 minutes (see inguinal hernia repair, page
16)

  (vi) If viability still doubtful then resect with end-to-end
anastomosis

 (vii) Decompress proximal bowel, either via NG tube or via
enterotomy with Foley catheter/Savage decompressor

(viii) Close enterotomy

7. Large bowel obstruction
    (i) Usually due to tumour, therefore if possible resect
   (ii) Either
      a. Perform end-to-end/end-to-side anastomosis with
protective colostomy or
      b. Bring out end colostomy for second stage operation
to rejoin bowel in continuity

8. Closure
    (i) Drain anastomosis region
   (ii) Close in layers

9. Postoperative management
    (i) Commence oral fluids when nasogastric aspirate
minimal and solids after passage of flatus per rectum
   (ii) Remove drain after 2–3 days

10. Complications
    (i) Early
      a. Prolonged ileus
      b. Aspiration pneumonia
      c. Anastomotic dehiscence
      d. Wound dehiscence
   (ii) Late
      a. Obstruction due to adhesions
      b. Incisional hernia
      c. Malabsorbtion with extensive resection

Hepatobiliary surgery

CHOLECYSTECTOMY

1. Indications
   - (i) *Calculous cholecystitis*
   - (ii) (Typhoid carrier)
   - (iii) (Carcinoma of the gall bladder)

2. Preoperative management
   - (i) Investigations
     - a. Ultrasound of gall bladder and bile ducts
     - b. Cholecystogram
     - c. If previously jaundiced — Liver function tests
       HBS Ag status
       Clotting screen
     - d. History of allergic reaction to X-ray contrast media
     - e. PTC/ERCP if jaundiced
   - (ii) The mortality of cholecystectomy in cirrhosis/portal hypertension is > 10%
   - (iii) Vitamin K if recently jaundiced
   - (iv) Antibiotics
     - a. Broad spectrum now generally accepted as one dose or three dose prophylaxis
     - b. Risk groups for infection in biliary surgery —
       > 70 years old
       Diabetic
       On steroids
       Jaundiced or recently jaundiced
       Common bile duct exploration
       Malignancy involving the biliary tree
       Common bile duct stones or stricture
   - (v) IVI (with 10% Mannitol infusion if jaundiced)
   - (vi) Nasogastric tube to deflate the stomach peroperatively

3. Pre-incision
   - (i) General anaesthetic (avoiding hepatotoxic agents such as halothane) and endotracheal intubation

(ii) Position
   Supine on an *X-ray operating table*
(iii) Skin preparation for an upper abdominal incision
4 Incision
   (i) Kochers right subcostal ⎫
   (ii) Right paramedian   ⎬ All equally acceptable
   (iii) Right upper transverse ⎭
5 Procedure
   (i) Full laparotomy with particular attention to:
       a. 'Saints Triad' — Gallstones
                            Hiatus hernia
                            Sigmoid diverticular disease
       b. Other causes of upper abdominal pain —
                            Peptic ulcer
                            Carcinoma of the stomach
                            Pancreatic carcinoma
                            Chronic pancreatitis
   (ii) Display the gall bladder
       a. Pack off the small bowel
       b. Retract the stomach and duodenum downwards
       c. Retract the liver upwards
   (iii) Retract the gall bladder laterally, held in a sponge
         holder or Moynihan gall bladder clamp and incise the
         peritoneum over the right free border of the lesser
         omentum
   (iv) Dissect out Calot's triangle bordered by
       a. Cystic duct inferiorly
       b. Cystic artery superiorly
       c. Common hepatic and right hepatic duct on the left
   (v) Ligate and divide the cystic artery in continuity
   (vi) Cannulate the cystic duct and aspirate bile for
        microbiological examination
   (vii) Perform the operative cholangiogram
       a. Remove all instruments and radio-opaque swabs
       b. Tilt the operating table 10° to the right (so the bile
          ducts do not overlie the spine)
       c. Stop the ventilator during X-ray exposure
       d. Take at least two films, after the injection of 2 and
          10 ml of contrast
   (viii) Points to establish on the operative cholangiogram
       a. *Clear visualisation of all the common bile and
          hepatic ducts with delineation of the anatomy*
       b. *No filling defects or strictures*
       c. *Free flow into the duodenum in all films*
       d. *Common bile duct not dilated greater than 11 mm*
       e. *Minimal retrograde flow of contrast into the
          pancreatic ducts*

(ix) If all these are established then withdraw the catheter and proceed

(x) Problems with peroperative cholangiography
   a. Introduction of air bubbles, mimicking radiolucent stones
   b. Spasm of the sphincter of Oddi
   c. Contrast in the duodenum obscuring the terminal common bile duct and ampulla

(xi) Complete the cholecystectomy
   a. Transfix and ligate the cystic duct within 1 cm of the common bile duct with an absorbable suture
   b. Divide the peritoneal reflection between the gall bladder and the liver and dissect the gall bladder out of its hepatic bed
   c. Use diathermy coagulation to control bleeding from the liver bed

(xii) Examine the gall bladder and gallstones. Send the gall bladder for histological examination to exclude co-existing malignancy

(xiii) Closure
   a. Absolute haemostasis — Cystic artery
   Gall bladder bed
   b. Suction drain to gall bladder bed
   c. T-tube brought out by a separate stab incision
   d. Close in layers

6. Postoperative management
   (i) Accurate measurements of drainage essential; suspect a significant leak if > 500 ml of bile is drained daily from the suction drain to the gall bladder bed
   (ii) Investigations
      a. Histology of gall bladder
      b. If T-tube present: T-tube cholangiogram to establish normal biliary flow and exclude retained stones prior to its removal

7. Complications
   (i) Early
      a. Biliary leak
      b. Ileus
      c. Wound infection
      d. Persistent jaundice with a retained stone
      e. Septicaemia
      f. Pancreatitis
   (ii) Late
      a. Cholangitis — Retained stone
      b. Biliary stricture

EXPLORATION OF THE COMMON BILE DUCT

1. Indications for choledochotomy/choledochoscopy
   (i) Abnormality noted on a preoperative or peroperative cholangiogram
   (ii) Obstructive jaundice not due to pancreatic or ampullary disease
   (iii) Palpable stones in the bile ducts
2. Factors in considering methods of choledochotomy

	Mortality (%)
Cholecystectomy	< 1
Supraduodenal choledochotomy	< 2
Transduodenal choledochotomy	< 4

   (i) Supraduodenal choledochotomy
      a. Place two stay sutures either side of the proposed 2 cm longitudinal incision in the common bile duct in the right free border of the lesser omentum
      b. Kocherise the duodenum to expose the full length of the common bile duct
      c. Incise the common bile duct longitudinally
      d. Close the choledochotomy with an absorbable suture over a latex T-tube brought out through a tunnel of greater omentum
3. Closure and postoperative management
   As for cholecystectomy (see page 104)

SPLENECTOMY

1. Indications
   (i) Trauma, if splenic preservation impractical (*Beware* associated left kidney injury)
   (ii) Haematological
      a. Haemolytic anaemia
      b. Myelofibrosis
      c. Leukaemia
   (iii) Not now commonly part of the staging of lymphoma
   (iv) Part of surgery for portal hypertension (see page 114) and pancreatic resection
2. Preoperative management
   (i) Trauma
      a. Resuscitate — Test urine for haematuria
                        Plain X-ray may show fractures of overlying ribs
                        Peritoneal lavage

      b. Catheterise
      c. Nasogastric tube
      d. IVI
   (ii) Haematological — Check
      a. Haemoglobin ⎫
      b. White cell count ⎬ Transfuse accordingly
      c. Platelet count ⎭
  (iii) Antibiotics
      In all cases broad spectrum and metronidazole
  (iv) Portal hypertension see page 114
3. Pre-incision
   (i) General anaesthetic with endotracheal intubation
  (ii) Position
      Supine
  (iii) Skin preparation for an upper abdominal incision
4. Incision
   (i) Left paramedian in trauma (better access to the rest of
      the abdomen) or
  (ii) Left Kocher subcostal
5. Procedure
   (i) Trauma — suck out all free blood and clots
  (ii) Place the left hand on the spleen and draw it down to
      divide the lieno renal ligament lying posteriorly
  (iii) Now deliver the spleen to the abdominal incision
  (iv) Examine the spleen; in trauma consider splenic repair
      and preservation
   (v) Ligate and divide
      a. Short gastric vessels
      b. Left gastro-epiploic vessel
         (Bury the stumps of these vessels on the greater
         curve of the stomach with an absorbable serosal
         suture to minimise the subsequent risk of ischaemic
         gastric perforation due to a ligature placed directly
         on the stomach)
  (vi) Gently separate the tail of the pancreas from the
      splenic vessels
  (vii) Clamp, separately divide and doubly ligate the splenic
      artery and splenic vein
 (viii) *Beware*
      a. *Tail of pancreas*
      b. *Splenic flexure of colon*
      c. *Left kidney and adrenal*
  (ix) Complete splenectomy by dividing the residual
      peritoneal attachments to the stomach and colon
   (x) Complete the laparotomy (see: laparotomy for
      abdominal trauma, page 179)

6. Closure
   (i) Meticulous haemostasis
   (ii) Peritoneal saline lavage
   (iii) Trauma — Place a suction drain to the tail of the pancreas
   (iv) Close in layers
7. Postoperative management
   (i) Remove
      a. Nasogastric tube when aspirate is minimal (24–48 hours)
      b. Drain when drainage is minimal (24–48 hours)
   (ii) Commence
      a. Oral fluids when flatus passed per rectum
      b. Long term pencillin V — 250 mg daily (to reduce the risk of opportunist infection, especially pneumococcus)
      c. Course of pneumococcal vaccine
8. Complications
   (i) Early
      a. Acute gastric dilatation
      b. Fundal ischaemia — Gastric perforation
                            Haematemesis
      c. Pancreatic fistula
      d. Portal vein thrombosis
      e. Reactionary haemorrhage from splenic vessels
   (ii) Late
      a. Increased infection — Pneumococcal
                               Viral
      b. Thrombocytosis

INTERNAL DRAINAGE OF A PANCREATIC PSEUDOCYST

1. Indications — Pseudocyst
   · (i) > 5 cm in diameter
   (ii) Symptomatic
   (iii) Infection
2. Preoperative management
   (i) Investigations
      a. Ultrasound
      b. Barium meal
      c. CT
      d. ERCP
   (ii) Antibiotics
      a. Broad spectrum
      b. Metronidazole
   (iii) Nasogastric tube
   (iv) IVI

3. Pre-incision
   (i) General anaesthetic with endotracheal intubation
   (ii) Position
       Supine on an X-ray table
   (iii) Skin preparation for an upper abdominal incision
4. Incision
   Upper midline
5. Procedure
   (i) Full laparotomy
   (ii) Insert a wide bore needle via the lesser or greater
        omentum into the cyst and aspirate cyst contents for
        a. Microbiological examination
        b. Cytological examination
        c. Amylase estimation
   (iii) Peroperative cystography can be performed by injecting
         20 ml of Hypaque into the cyst cavity
   (iv) Perform an anterior longitudinal gastrotomy of about
        8 cm in length. Achieve haemostasis at the gastric
        edges
   (v) Make a 5–6 cm linear incision in the posterior wall of
       the stomach to enter the pseudocyst
   (vi) Suck out the fluid and remove any solid debris
   (vii) Oversew the edges of the cyst gastrotomy with an
         absorbable suture
   (viii) Close the anterior gastrotomy in two layers
6. Closure
   (i) No drains
   (ii) Close in layers
7. Alternative method of drainage
   (i) Cyst lying adjacent to head of pancreas: cyst-
       duodenostomy
   (ii) Cyst lying in transverse mesocolon: cyst-jejunostomy
        Roux-en-Y
   (iii) Cyst lying at the tail of the pancreas: resect
8. Postoperative management
   (i) Remove nasogastric tube when aspirate is minimal
   (ii) Commence oral fluids when flatus is passed per rectum
   (iii) Investigation repeat ultrasound/CT
9. Complications
   (i) Early
       a. Secondary haemorrhage from vessels of the cyst
          wall
       b. Recurrent cyst
       c. Fistula from anastomotic leak
   (ii) Late
        Recurrent cyst

'TRIPLE BYPASS' OPERATION FOR CARCINOMA OF THE HEAD OF THE PANCREAS

1. Preoperative management
   (i) Investigations
      a. Diagnostic — Liver function tests
                      Ultrasound of biliary tree and pancreas
                      Percutaneous transhepatic
                      cholangiogram
                      ERCP with pancreatic cytology
                      CT
      b. Therapeutic — Clotting screen; if the prothrombin
                      time is abnormal then give parenteral
                      Vitamin K
      c. Preoperative percutaneous biliary decompression has
         not been shown to improve operative mortality and
         morbidity, and carries a significant morbidity
   (ii) Antibiotics — broad spectrum and metronidazole
   (iii) IVI with a 20% Mannitol infusion peroperatively to
         protect the renal tubules by osmotic diuresis
   (iv) Catheterise
   (v) Nasogastric tube
2. Pre-incision
   (i) General anaesthesia with endotracheal intubation
   (ii) Position
        Supine on X-ray table (if percutaneous
        cholangiography is required)
   (iii) Skin preparation for an upper abdominal incision
3. Incision
   Upper midline
4. Procedure
   (i) Full laparotomy
      a. Assess the resectability of the tumour
      b. Evidence of metastases (liver, pre-aortic nodes,
         peritoneum)
      c. Tumour size and fixation
   (ii) If the tumour is considered to be unresectable then
        proceed to a palliative bypass procedure after biopsying
        the tumour
5. Method of biopsy
   (i) Trucut needle
      a. Transduodenally
      b. Direct
   (ii) Open
      a. Pancreas
      b. Regional nodes
6. Cholecystojejunostomy
   (i) Decompress the distended tense gall bladder by

fashioning a fundal purse-string suture and inserting a gall
bladder trochar and suction cannula through a
cholecystostomy within the purse-string
   (ii) Cholangiography may be performed at this stage
   (iii) Anastomose the gall bladder fundus in two layers to an
        available loop of proximal jejunum
7. Gastroenterostomy
   Anastomose the stomach side-to-side to a loop of jejunum
   proximal to the cholecyst-jejunostomy
8. Entero-enterostomy
   Anastomose a segment of jejunum between the
   gastrojejunostomy and the cholecyst-jejunostomy side-to-side
   to a segment of jejunum distal to the cholecyst-jejunostomy in
   two layers
9. Purpose of bypass procedures
   (i) Gastro-jejunostomy
       Bypasses duodenal obstruction by the pancreatic tumour
   (ii) Cholecyst-jejunostomy
        Maintains biliary drainage (unless the tumour invades as
        far as the cystic duct which may enter the common bile
        duct low down)
   (iii) Entero-enterostomy
        Diverts small bowel content away from the cholecyst-
        jejunostomy reducing the risk of cholangitis
10. Closure
    (i) Meticulous haemostasis in the jaundiced patient
    (ii) Drain anastomoses
    (iii) Close in layers
11. Postoperative management
    (i) Aspirate nasogastric tube until the aspirate is minimal
        and commence oral fluids at the passage of flatus per
        rectum
    (ii) Investigations
        a. Histology of tumour
        b. Liver function tests
        c. Renal function
12. Complications
    (i) Early
        a. Septicaemia
        b. Cholangitis
        c. Ileus
        d. Obstruction of anastomoses with oedema
    (ii) Late
        a. Recurrent jaundice — 20%
        b. Cholangitis
        c. Tumour spread
        d. Gastric outflow obstruction with tumour spread —
           15%

PRINCIPLES OF HEPATIC RESECTION
1. Indications
    (i) Hepatic tumour
        a. Benign — 'Pill' tumour
                    Adenoma
        b. Malignant — Primary — Hepatoblastoma
                                 Hepatocellular carcinoma
                      Secondary (see Table below)
    (ii) Hepatic cyst
        a. Congenital — Leave
        b. Hydatid — Only treat if symptomatic
    (iii) Trauma
        a. (80% of serious liver injuries have concommitant serious injury to other viscera, see laparotomy for abdominal trauma, page 179)
        b. Liver + duodenum/pancreas — 50%
        c. Liver + colon — 20%

Place of surgery in the management of hepatic secondaries
Resection surgery is worthwhile for
    (i) Colorectal primary
    (ii) Symptomatic carcinoid (consider embolisation)
    (iii) Others; Wilms, renal adenocarcinoma

Liver metastasis from colorectal primary

	Mean survival, months (no treatment)	Mean survival, months (hepatic resection)
Stage 1 — Solitary metastasis	16	24
Stage 2 — Culster of metastases	10	17
Stage 3 — Scattered metastases	3	—

Hepatic artery embolisation/ligation for endocrine secreting liver metastases
    (i) Never in the presence of jaundice
    (ii) Needs preoperative angiography
        a. Show pathology
        b. Show anatomy
    (iii) Infuse dextrose 10% and insulin during the procedure to protect hepatocytes
    (iv) Needs 48 hours of parenteral antibiotic prophylaxis
    (v) Best results in carcinoid

2. Investigation in hepatic malignancy
    (i)   Liver function tests
    (ii) 5 gamma glutamyl transferase
    (iii) Alpha-feto protein
    (iv) Gut hormone screen
    (v)   Liver isotope scan (sulphur-colloid)
    (vi) Liver ultrasound
    (vii) Hepatic artery and portal vein angiography
    (viii) Inferior vena cavagram
    (ix) CT
    (x)   Biopsy
          a. Fine needle aspiration ⎫
          b. True cut biopsy   ⎬ May seed tumour
          c. Laparoscopic   ⎭
    (xi) Cholangiography
          PTC
3. Anatomical and physiological factors
    (i)   The 'surgical' right and left lobes of the liver are
          determined by the vascular anatomy of the portal veins
          and hepatic artery. The line of division lies within the
          anatomical right lobe, lateral to the falciform ligament
          and follows the line between the gall bladder bed and
          the IVC. The only large structure expected in this plane
          is the middle hepatic vein
    (ii) Preoperatively correct
          a. Serum albumin
          b. Clotting
          c. Sepsis
    (iii) Peroperatively
          a. Needs intensive cardiovascular monitoring
          b. Access for rapid transfusion (beware air embolism
             and the effects of caval compression)
4. Principles of hepatic lobe resection
    (i)   Dissect out the porta hepatis, ligate and divide the
          branch of the hepatic artery, hepatic duct and portal
          vein to the relevant lobe
    (ii) The division between the devitalised lobe and the rest
          of the liver is now apparent
    (iii) Divide the liver by the 'finger fracture' technique,
          ligating and dividing any vessels crossing between the
          two parts of the liver, divide and transfix hepatic vein
5. Principles of surgery for liver trauma
    Object is to control haemorrhage and remove all dead tissue
    (i)   Good access — right thoracoabdominal incision
    (ii) Pringles manoeuvre; compressing the right free border of
          the lesser omentum with the hepatic artery and portal
          vein

(iii) Control of the vena cava above and below the liver
(iv) Aims of surgery
    a. Resect all devitalised liver
    b. Haemostasis
       Direct suture of bleeding vessels (*avoid tight sutures*)
       Hepatic artery ligation
       Omental graft
       Pack uncontrollable bleeding
    c. Prevent bile leakage
       Adequate drainage of all damaged areas
6. Postoperative management
   (i) Check albumin daily, may need replacements for up to three weeks
  (ii) Check blood sugar, may fall dramatically in the first 48 hours
 (iii) Bleeding problems
    a. Reactionary
    b. Vitamin K deficiency
7. Complications of liver surgery
   (i) Early
    a. Jaundice
    b. Hypoalbuminaemia
    c. Hypoglycaemia
    d. Sepsis — Cholangitis
             Septicaemia
             Abscess — Intrahepatic
                     Subphrenic
    e Upper GI haemorrhage
    f. Biliary fistula
    g. Renal failure ('hepato-renal' syndrome in obstructive jaundice)
    h. Adult respiratory distress syndrome
  (ii) Late
    a. Portal hypertension
    b. Biliary stricture
    c. Haemobilia
8. Factors in morbidity and mortality
   (i) Age
  (ii) Previous biliary surgery
 (iii) Biliary infection
 (iv) Biliary obstruction
  (v) Cirrhosis
 (vi) Associated pathology
(vii) Extent of liver trauma and associated injuries (chest and head)

PRINCIPLES OF SURGERY FOR PORTAL HYPERTENSION

1. Classification
   (i) Prehepatic (congenital portal malformation, portal vein thrombosis or compression)
   (ii) Hepatic — (Cirrhosis, schistosomiasis)
   (iii) Posthepatic (Budd Chiari, tricuspid incompetence)
2. Complications of portal hypertension
   (i) Upper GI bleeding
      a. Decreased clotting factors
      b. Varices
      c. Increased incidence of peptic ulcer
   (ii) Hypersplenism with thrombocytopenia
   (iii) Ascites
      a. Increased portal pressure
      b. Decreased serum albumin
      c. Hepatic lymphatic obstruction
   (iv) Hepatic encephalopathy
3. Control of bleeding varices
   (i) Investigations
      a. Emergency ⎰ Endoscopy — Diagnostic
                    ⎱   Allows sclerotherapy
                      Clotting screen
      b. Electrolytes
      c. Liver function tests
      d. HB SAg status
      e. Alpha feto protein
      f. Portogram — Direct splenic puncture
                     (allows portal manometry)
                     Venous phase of coeliac axis
                     arteriogram
   (ii) Conservative
      a. Pharmocological — Pitressin
                           Somatostatin
                           Propranolol
      b. Tamponade — Sengstaken — Blakemore tube
                     St James tube
   (iii) Veno occlusion
      a. Endoscopic sclerotherapy
      b. Transhepatic radiological embolisation
      c. Surgery — Oesophageal transection
                   Oesophageal stapling
   (iv) Surgical decompression
4. Indications for surgery
   (i) Uncontrollable bleeding from varices

(ii) Elective
  a. Previous severe bleed
  b. Good liver cell function
  c. Good clinical condition
  d. Social — Age of patient (younger better)
     Distance to travel if bleeds again

5. Oesophageal transection
  (i) Use abdominal approach
  (ii) Mobilise lower oesophagus and separate the vagi away from the oesophagus
  (iii) Pass a sling around the oesophagus
  (iv) Perform a gastrotomy and introduce a circular stapling gun
  (v) Ligate the cardia around the neck of the open stapling gun, close the anvil and fire the gun
  (vi) Gently release the stapling gun, having transected the cardia with reanastomosis of the oesophagus to the stomach by a ring of staples

6. Portal decompression
  (i) Either
    a. Emergency
    b. Electively
    c. No place as prophylaxis for varices found incidentally as 60% do not bleed severely
  (ii) Portocaval
    a. End-to-side
    b. > 50% encephalopathy
  (iii) Spleno-renal
    a. End-to-side with splenectomy
    b. > 40% encephalopathy
  (iv) Mesocaval
    a. Side-to-side with a Dacron graft
    b. High incidence of graft thrombosis
  (v) Distal spleno-renal
    a. Selectively decompresses the venous drainage of the cardia
    b. Reduced incidence of encephalopathy

7. Mortality
  (i) Emergency surgery
    a. Oesophageal transection — 40%
    b. Decompression — 50%
  (ii) Due to
    a. Electrolyte problems
    b. Aspiration
    c. Acute renal failure
    d. Hepatic failure
    e. Encephalopathy
    f. Disseminated intravascular coagulation

Colorectal surgery

PRINCIPLES OF BOWEL PREPARATION FOR COLORECTAL SURGERY

Never on totally obstructed bowel
  Only with great care from above on partially obstructed bowel with assistance of enemata
  All need broad spectrum and metronidazole antibiotic prophylaxis
1 Traditional
    (i) Commence on the 5th preoperative day: oral magnesium sulphate and a disposable enema
   (ii) 4th and 3rd preoperative day: low residue diet and magnesium sulphate with daily soap and water enemata
   (iii) 2nd and last preoperative day: fluid diet and castor oil with daily soap and water enemata
   (iv) Comment
      a. Requires admission 5–6 days before surgery
      b. Cleanliness of bowel mucosa not as good as methods 2 and 3
      c. Relatively safe in partial obstruction
2 Laxative method
    (i) Commence on the day before surgery
   (ii) Give 75–150 g Mannitol in 300–1000 ml of water orally or 1–2 sachets of Picolax and two high enemata on the day before surgery
   (iii) Comment
      a. Bowel cleanliness not as good a method 3
      b. May produce considerable gaseous distension
3 Whole gut irrigation
    (i) Commence on the day before surgery
   (ii) Give an oral pre-med of
      a. Metoclopramide   10 mg
      b. Diazepam   15 mg
      c. Magnesium sulphate 5 mg
   (iii) Pass a soft nasogastric tube as far as the duodenum under X-ray control

(iv) Irrigate with normal saline (at body temperature, 37°C) at 2–4 litres per hour until the anal effluent runs crystal clear

(v) Comment
   a. Gives the cleanest bowel preparation
   b. May cause severe water and electrolyte imbalance, especially in the elderly

(vi) Therefore, needs electrolyte check before and after the procedure beware congestive cardiac failure with fluid overload and avoid in poor myocardial state

4. Bowel preparation for emergency colonic surgery
   (i) Irrigation from below prior to surgery
   (ii) Irrigate the colon on the table via a caecostomy tube

APPENDICECTOMY

1. Preoperative management
   (i) Investigations
      a. White cell count
      b. Urinalysis, exclude UTI
   (ii) If dehydrated due to vomiting, then rehydrate with saline
   (iii) Antibiotic prophylaxis
      a. Metronidazole by suppository
      b. Evidence of perforation: add parenteral broad spectrum antibiotic

2. Pre-incision
   (i) General anaesthesia and endotracheal intubation
   (ii) Position
      Supine
   (iii) Skin preparation for an incision in the right iliac fossa, but prepare all the abdomen

3. Incision
   Grid iron (right iliac fossa over MacBurney's point)

4. Procedure
   (i) Deepen the incision by splitting the muscle layers in the line of their fibres.
   (ii) As the peritoneum is opened, remove a sample of peritoneal fluid for microbiological examination
   (iii) Withdraw the caecum gently, locate and deliver the appendix
   (iv) Place haemostatic forceps across the appendix mesentery and divide it, ligating the vessels
   (v) Place a pursestring suture around the taenia coli, 2 cm from the base of the appendix
   (vi) Place crushing forceps just distal to the base of the appendix and ligate the base of the appendix with an absorbable ligature just proximal to this

(vii) Remove the appendix flush with the caecal side of the crushing forceps. Send for histological examination

(viii) Invaginate the appendix stump in the caecum and tie the pursestring to bury the stump

(ix) Perform a local peritoneal toilet

5. Problem
   (i) Not appendicitis, exclude
      a. Mesenteric adenitis
      b. Right tubo-ovarian pathology
      c. Cholecystitis
      d. Ileitis — Yersinia
                    Crohn's
      e. Carcinoma of the caecum
   (ii) Incidental Meckel's diverticulum
      a. Normal — Leave
      b. Inflamed — Remove
   (iii) Appendicitis in the presence of Crohn's disease
      a. Ileal Crohn's, perform appendicectomy
      b. Caecal Crohn's, leave appendix and drain the peritoneum

6. Closure
   (i) Close in layers
   (ii) No drains
   (iii) If the wound is severely contaminated then irrigate with antiseptic solution

7. Postoperative management
   (i) Investigate histology of appendix
   (ii) Rare problems
      a. Appendix carcinoid — No further treatment necessary
      b. Adenocarcinoma — Needs a right hemicolectomy
   (iii) Microbiological results from peritoneal fluid
   (iv) Continue metronidazole suppositories for 48 hours

8. Complications
   (i) Early
      a. Infection — Peritonitis
                      Septicaemia
                      Wound
                      Abscess — Pelvic
                                 Subphrenic
      b. Ileus
      c. Haemorrhage from appendix mesentery (usually reactionary)
      d. (Portal pyaemia)
      e. (Fistula)
   (ii) Late
      a. Adhesions — Small bowel obstruction
                     Fallopian tube obstruction

ILEOSTOMY

1. Indications
   (i) Total colectomy
   (ii) Defunctioning
   To protect ileo-anal anastomosis
2. Preoperative management
   (i) Examine the patient standing, sitting and lying flat to determine the appropriate site in the right iliac fossa for the stoma. Never in a skin fold or near a scar. Introduce the patient to the stoma therapist and encourage psychological support
   (ii) Investigations — Those appropriate to the pathology
       a. Ulcerative colitis
       b. Toxic megacolon
       c. Familial polyposis coli
   (iii) IVI
   (iv) Catheter   } For total
   (v) Nasogastric tube } colectomy
   (vi) Broad spectrum and metronidazole antibiotic prophylaxis
3. Pre-incision
   (i) General anaesthestic with endotracheal intubation
   (ii) Position
       a. Lithotomy — Trendelenberg with Lloyd Davis stirrups for panproctocolectomy
       b. Supine for total colectomy with rectal preservation
   (iii) Skin preparation of all of abdomen including perineum for panproctocolectomy
4. Incision
   Left paramedian
5. Procedure
   (i) After the colon ± rectum have been mobilised and resected, usually with the last 10–20 cm of terminal ileum, divide the mesentery preserving all branches proximal to the terminal ileocolic vessels and examine the cut end of ileum to ensure bleeding and viability
   (ii) Cut out a 3 cm disc of skin at the designated ileostomy site, and a further disc of all layers deep to this including the peritoneum
   (iii) Pass the ileal end through the ileostomy hole to protrude by 5 cm and close the lateral space between mesentery and parietal peritoneum with a continuous absorbable suture
6. Alternative — Extraperitoneal method
   (i) Do not open the peritoneum at the ileostomy hole

(ii) Pass the end of the ileum under the peritoneum lateral to the caecal reflexion and burrow it extraperitoneally to the ileostomy hole. Now there is no lateral space to close
7. Closure
   (i) Close the abdominal wound in layers with appropriate drains for the procedure undertaken
   (ii) Fashion the ileostomy spout by everting the last 2–3 cm of ileum and place several interrupted absorbable sutures between ileum and skin around its circumference
   (iii) Place an ileostomy bag over the stoma
8. Postoperative management
   (i) Histological examination of the resected specimen
   (ii) Control
      a. Allow a normal diet but encourage the patient to avoid any food which upsets the stoma
      b. Usually works after each meal
      c. If too liquid, use loperamide
   Complications
   (i) Skin excoriation
   (ii) Retraction
   (iii) Prolapse
   (iv) Small bowel obstruction
      a. Adhesions
      b. Lateral space herniation

TRANSVERSE COLOSTOMY

1. Indications
   (i) Elective
   Defunction the descending colon and rectum
   (ii) Emergency
   As the first stage of treatment for a complete obstruction of the distal colon
2. Preoperative management
   (i) Fully informed consent, explain how the colostomy functions and (if possible) introduce the patient to the stoma therapist to explain about stoma care
   (ii) Investigations — Those relevant to the pathology
      a. Abdominal plain X-rays
      b. Sigmoidoscopy
      c. Colonoscopy | Except in perforated
      d. Barium enema | diverticular disease
   (iii) Preparation
      a. Bowel preparation if not obstructed (see page 116)
      b. If obstructed, correct — Anaemia
                          Fluid and electrolyte balance

     (iv) Broad spectrum and metronidazole antibiotic prophylaxis
     (v) Nasogastric tube
     (vi) IVI
    (vii) Catheter, if obstructed

3. Pre-incision
     (i) General anaesthesia with endotracheal intubation
    (ii) Position
       Supine
    (iii) Skin preparation of whole of abdomen

4. Incision
   10 cm transverse incision in the right upper quadrent

5. Procedure
     (i) Assess the intra-peritoneal pathology by as full a laparotomy as possible via the incision
    (ii) Locate and withdraw the transverse colon (identified by the attachment of greater omentum)
    (iii) Locate a point on the colon proximal to the middle colic artery and detach the omentum from the colon at this point
    (iv) Open a window at an avascular point in the mesocolon at this point and pass a glass or plastic rod through this hole
     (v) Wrap the redundant omentum around the proximal and distal limbs of the colon
    (vi) Close the wound in layers around the prepared transverse colon with the greater omentum plugging the corners at each end. The rod now sits outside the wound
    (vii) Once the wound is closed around the colon, open the colon along a taenia and suture the mucosa of the colon to the skin edges with interrupted absorbable sutures
   (viii) Secure the rod with a length of rubber tubing over each end and place a colostomy bag over the stoma

6. Postoperative management
     (i) Commence oral fluids next day and colostomy training as soon as possible
    (ii) Remove the securing rod after 3–4 days

7. Complications
     (i) Colostomy retraction
    (ii) Colostomy prolapse
    (iii) Parastomal herniation
    (iv) Ischaemia of colostomy
     (v) Stomal stenosis
    (vi) Stomal ulceration
    (vii) Stomal obstruction
   (viii) Faecal overflow into distal limb rendering defunctioning ineffective

CLOSURE OF TRANSVERSE COLOSTOMY

1. Preoperative management
    (i) Distal limb barium enema (to assess resolution
        of pathology or integrity of anastomosis)
    (ii) Preparation of bowel including distal limb washouts
    (iii) Nasogastric tube optional
    (iv) IVI
    (v) Broad spectrum and metronidazole antibiotic
        prophylaxis
2. Pre-incision
    (i) Pick up the collar of parastomal skin in tissue holding
        forceps
    (ii) Mobilise colostomy by incising directly through all
        layers to the peritoneum
    (iii) *Beware*
        a. Perforating the colon, especially at the junction with
           the rectus sheath
        b. Perforation of an insinuated loop of small bowel
    (iv) Excise the collar of skin and fibrous tissue from the
        colon by sharp dissection
    (v) Close the colon in two layers and return to the
        peritoneum
3. Closure
    (i) Intraperitoneal drain to colonic closure
    (ii) Close in layers
4. Postoperative management
    (i) Commence oral fluids when flatus passed per rectum
    (ii) Remove the drain when faeces are passed
5. Complications
    (i) Stenosis at colostomy closure (rare)
    (ii) Leakage
        a. Faecal peritonitis
        b. Abscess
        c. Fistula (especially if closed by the extra peritoneal
           method)

OPERATIONS FOR COLORECTAL CARCINOMA — GENERAL PRINCIPLES

1. Preoperative management
    (i) Investigations
        a. Haemoglobin, correct anaemia if present
        b. Barium enema   ⎫ Exclude multiple primary
        c. Colonoscopy with biopsy ⎭ tumours
        d. IVP to exclude ureteric involvement

    (ii) Full bowel preparation
   (iii) Broad spectrum with metronidazole antibiotic
       prophylaxis
   (iv) IVI
    (v) Nasogastric tube
   (vi) Catheter
2. Pre-incision
  General anaesthesia with endotracheal intubation
3. Procedure
    (i) Full laparotomy
   (ii) Assess the tumour operability
      a. Site and proximal obstruction
      b. Fixity (*avoid undue handling*)
      c. Spread — Locally
              Nodes
              Liver
              Peritoneum
   (iii) Specific operation (see pages 124–132)
4. Postoperative management
    (i) Commence oral fluids at the passage of flatus per
      rectum/stoma
   (ii) Continue prophylactic antibiotics parenterally for two
      further doses
   (iii) Remove drain at the first passage of a solid stool
5. Complications
    (i) Early
      a. Anastomosis — Stricture
                 Breakdown with leakage
      b. Infection   — Abscess
                 Peritonitis
                 Wound infection
                 Septicaemia
                 (portal pyaemia)
      c. Haemorrhage — Reactionary
   (ii) Late

      a. Obstruction — Adhesions
                 Anastomosis — Stricture
                            Local
                            recurrence
      b. Tumour recurrence — Locally
                     Metastases — Liver
                              Peritoneum
                     New primary

RIGHT HEMICOLECTOMY

(See general principles, page 122)
1. Pre-incision
    (i) Position
        Supine with 20° tilt of the table to the left; the surgeon
        stands on the left side of the patient
    (ii) Skin preparation of all of abdomen
2. Incision
    Right paramedian
3. Procedure
    (i) Ligate/clamp the bowel proximally and distally to the
        tumour to reduce intraluminal spread
    (ii) Divide the peritoneum 2 cm lateral and parallel to the
        colon from the caecum to the hepatic flexure. Mobilise
        the ascending colon medially
    (iii) *Beware*
        a. *Right kidney*
        b. *Duodenum*
        c. *Right ureter*
        d. *Right gonadal vessels*
    (iv) Elevate the bowel to expose the origin of the ileo-colic
        artery: ligate and divide
        a. Right branches of middle colic vessels
        b. Right colic vessels
        c. Ileo-colic vessels
        d. Vessels to last 30 cm of ileum
    (v) Place soft bowel clamps on ileum, 30 cm from ileo-colic
        valve and at the junction of the proximal and middle
        third of the transverse colon
    (vi) Place crushing bowel clamps 2–3 cm within the soft
        bowel clamps on the bowel to be resected
    (vii) Divide the bowel flush with the crushing clamps and
        remove the specimen
    (viii) Anastomose the ileum end-to-end or end-to-side with
        the transverse colon in two layers
4. Problems
    (i) Multiple secondaries
        Perform local resection of tumour to reduce the chances
        of mechanical obstruction
    (ii) Irresectable tumour
        Ileo-transverse anastomosis
5. Closure
    (see general principles, page 123)
    (i) Corrugated drain to anastomosis area
    (ii) Close in layers

LEFT HEMICOLECTOMY

1. Preoperative management
   advise the patient of the possible necessity for a
   defunctioning colostomy to protect a colonic anastomosis
   (see general principles, page 122)
2. Pre-incision
   (i) Position
       a. Supine with 20°C tilt on the table to the right
       b. Surgeon standing on the patient's right
   (ii) Skin preparation of all of abdomen, towel up for a left
       paramedian incision
3. Incision
   Left paramedian
4. Procedure
   (i) Ligate or clamp the bowel proximally and distally to the
       tumour to reduce intraluminal spread as a result of
       operative manoeuvres
   (ii) Incise the peritoneum 2 cm lateral to the sigmoid colon
       and continue upwards parallel to the descending colon
       including the splenic flexure
   (iii) Divide the peritoneal reflection between the splenic
       flexure and the spleen
   (iv) *Beware*
       a. *Spleen*
       b. *Tail of pancreas*
       c. *Left kidney*
       d. *Left ureter*
       e. *Left gonadal vessels*
   (v) Elevate the colon medially to display the inferior
       mesenteric vessels
   (vi) Ligate and divide
       a. Inferior mesenteric artery, flush with the aorta
       b. Inferior mesenteric vein
       c. Left branch of middle colic vessels
       d. Marginal vessels at mid transverse colon
   (vii) Place soft bowel clamps at the junction of mid-third
       and distal-third of transverse colon and distal sigmoid
       colon. Place crushing clamps 2–3 cm within these soft
       bowel clamps
   (viii) Divide the bowel flush with the crushing clamps and
       remove the specimen for histological examination
   (ix) (It may be necessary to mobilise the hepatic flexure in
       order to perform the colo-colonic anastomosis without
       tension)
   (x) Perform an end-to-end colo-colonic anastomosis in two
       layers

5. Problems
   (i) Irresectable tumour — defunctioning transverse colostomy
   (ii) Resectable tumour with multiple metastases — limited bowel resection with end-to-end anastomosis to reduce the risk of mechanical obstruction
   (iii) Large bowel obstruction due to tumour or inadequate bowel preparation
        Perform left hemicolectomy as above but protect the anastomosis with a defunctioning transverse colostomy
6. Closure
   (i) Corrugated drain to anastomosis
   (ii) Wash out any faecal spillage with warm saline (antiseptic optional)
   (iii) Close in layers
7. Postoperative management
   investigate using distal limb barium enema prior to closure of defunctioning colostomy
   (See general principles, page 123)

ANTERIOR RESECTION OF THE RECTUM

1. Indications
   (i) Rectal carcinoma between 8 cm from anus and the recto-sigmoid junction
   (ii) Small resectable primary low rectal malignancy with metastases (avoids colostomy)
2. Preoperative management
   Warn the patient of the possible need for a colostomy (defunctioning transverse or end colostomy if an abdomino-perineal excision becomes necessary)
   (See general principles, page 122)
3. Pre-incision
   (i) Position
       Lithotomy — Trendelenberg in Lloyd Davis stirrups allows access to the anus for either abdomino-perineal excision if necessary or a low rectal anastomosis using a circular stapling gun
   (ii) Skin preparation of whole of abdomen for a left paramedian incision
4. Incision
   Long left paramedian
5. Procedure
   (i) Mobilise the splenic flexure of the colon. Continue by dividing the peritoneum 2 cm lateral to the descending colon down to the sigmoid mesentery

(ii) Ligate and divide the inferior mesenteric vessels and their branches below the level of mid sigmoid.
Continue the peritoneal incision onto both leaves of sigmoid mesentery to envelope the rectum

(iii) *Beware left ureter as it crosses the bifurcation of the common iliac artery*

(iv) Mobilise the rectum: divide
    a. The mesorectum posteriorly
    b. Lateral ligaments of the rectum

(v) *Beware both ureters in the pelvis* as they lie adjacent to the lateral rectal ligaments
Ligate the stumps of the lateral rectal ligaments

(vi) The rectum is now mobilised and can be delivered into the abdomen. The tumour should be palpable

(vii) Place two soft bowel clamps, one across mid sigmoid colon and the other at least 3–4 cm below the tumour across the distal rectum. Place crushing clamps across the bowel 1–2 cm within the soft clamps

(viii) Divide the bowel flush with the crushing clamps and remove the specimen

(ix) Perform the anastomosis between the mobilised descending/sigmoid colon and distal rectum with either a single layer of interrupted sutures or using a circular stapling gun passed per anum

6. Closure
    (i) Place a corrugated drain down to the anastomosis brought out via a separate stab incision
    (ii) Doubt about the viability of the anastomosis then a defunctioning transverse colostomy to protect it (see closure of transverse colostomy, page 120)
    (iii) Close in layers

7. Postoperative management
    (i) Remove the pelvic drain after the passage of solid faeces through the anastomosis
    (ii) Complications
        a. Early — Acute retention of urine
        b. Late — Anastomotic stricture — Treat by rectal dilatation
        (see general principles page 123)

ABDOMINO-PERINEAL EXCISION OF THE RECTUM

1. Indications
    (i) Carcinoma of the rectum within 6 cm of the anus
    (ii) Carcinoma of the anus
        (see general principles, page 122)

2. Preoperative management
Fully informed consent about the nature of the colostomy,
introduce the patient to the stoma therapist and mark the
site of the colostomy midway between the anterior superior
iliac spine and the umbilicus in the standing, sitting and
lying position, the final position being a compromise of the
three, avoiding skin creases
3. Pre-incision
    (i) Position
        Lithotomy — Trendelenberg with Lloyd Davis stirrups.
        The shoulders and sacrum should be well supported
   (ii) Skin preparation of all of abdomen and perineum. Towel
        up each leg separately and cover the genitals, leaving
        the perineum and abdomen exposed
  (iii) Position of operators
        a. Abdominal operator on the left
        b. Perineal operating sitting, facing the perineum
   (iv) Perineal operator
        Pursestring with a stout silk suture around the anus and
        tie off to reduce faecal spillage
4. Incision
Commence with a low left paramedian incision
5. Procedure:
Abdominal operator
    (i) Full laparotomy, with special regard to the tumour (see
        general principles, page 122). If the tumour is resectable
        then allow the perineal operator to commence
   (ii) Pack away the small bowel towards the right
        hypochondrium and retract the wound edges with a
        self retaining retractor (eg Goligher's)
  (iii) Mobilise the sigmoid colon by dividing the peritoneum
        1–2 cm lateral to it down as far as the rectum
   (iv) *Beware the left ureter as it crosses the bifurcation of
        the common iliac artery*
    (v) Divide the right leaf of the pelvic mesocolon as it
        descends around the upper third of the rectum
   (vi) *Beware the adjacent right ureter*
  (vii) Ligate and divide the inferior mesenteric vessels
 (viii) Select the level of transection on the descending colon
        and clean the appendices epiploicae off the bowel.
        Place a soft bowel clamp across the bowel and a
        crushing clamp 2 cm distal to this
   (ix) Divide the bowel flush with the crushing clamp
    (x) Mobilise the rectum by dividing the posterior
        mesorectum
   (xi) *Beware the presacral plexus*
  (xii) Ligate and divide the lateral ligaments of the rectum
        containing the middle rectal vessels
 (xiii) *Beware the ureters lying laterally*

(xiv) In the male
    a. Divide the fascia of Denonvilliers anteriorly
    b. *Beware the seminal vesicles anteriorly*
(xv) In the female incise the posterior wall of the vagina
    jointly with the perineal operator

6 Procedure:
Perineal operator
  (i) Incision
    Elliptical commencing at the coccyx and passing 2 cm
    lateral to the anal verge and finishing:
    a. Male — At the pineral body
    b. Female — At the posterior wall of the vagina
  (ii) Place a self retaining retractor within the wound
  (iii) Deepen the incision
    a. Posteriorly to the mesorectum to meet the abdominal
      operator through Waldeyer's fascia
    b. Hook the index finger of the left hand around the
      posterior edge of the levator ani muscles and divide
      the muscles with scissors immediately lateral to the
      index finger, clamping and ligating bleeding points
  (iv) Retracting on the anus with a strong pair of tissue
    holding forceps commence the anterior dissection
    a. Male — Palpate the urethral catheter lying in the
             bulbar urethra, carefully dissect upwards in
             the plane of the fascia of Denonvilliers using
             scissors
    b. Female — Excise the posterior wall of the vagina to
             the posterior fornix
  (v) The rectum is now completely free and is delivered to
    the perineal operator with the upper end clamped off by
    the crushing clamp

7. Closure
  (i) Abdominal operator
    a. Create a 3 cm diameter all layers circular incision at
      the predetermined site for the colostomy. Deliver the
      mobilised free end of the descending colon through
      this incision
    b. No intra-abdominal drains
    c. Close the pelvic peritoneum over the defect
    d. Close the abdominal wound in layers
    e. Fashion the end colostomy using 8–10 interrupted
      absorbable mucocutaneous sutures
    f. Place a colostomy bag over the stoma
  (ii) Perineal operator
    a. Absolute haemostasis is very important
    b. Place a suction drain into the pelvic defect
    c. Close the levator ani muscles
    d. Close the perineal skin

8. Problems
    (i) Continuing bleeding
        a. Moderate bleeding: pack the defect with a polythene sheet held in place by a long gauze roll pack which can be gradually shortened as the wound is allowed to granulate
        b. Severe bleeding: consider ligation of the internal iliac vessels by the abdominal operator or radiological embolisation
9. Postoperative management
    (i) Remove the perineal drain when drainage is minimal
    (ii) Remove the catheter after 3–4 days. Haematuria after this procedure is very common as a result of blunt trauma to the bladder
    (iii) Commence colostomy training as soon as possible continuing psychological support
10. Complications
    (i) Early
        a. Infection   — Wound infection
                            Pelvic abscess
        b. Colostomy — (See transverse colostomy, page 120)
        c. Genito-urinary — Haematuria
                            Retention, especially in males. 10% is permanent due to either prostatism or neurological damage during the procedure
                            Impotence
                            Fistula — Uretero-perineal
                                    Urethro-perineal
    (ii) Late
        a. Tumour recurrence — see general principles page 123
        b. Pelvic recurrence may present as sciatica

HARTMANN'S OPERATION

1. Indications
    (i) Obstructing carcinoma at the recto-sigmoid junction, especially in the elderly
    (ii) Perforation of a sigmoid diverticulum with gross inflammatory change of the adjacent colon
    (iii) First stage of surgery for sigmoid volvulus
2. Preoperative management
    (i) This operation is performed in the emergency situation on unprepared bowel so warn the patient of the subsequent colostomy
    (ii) Resuscitate
        a. Correct — Electrolytes
                    Anaemia

b. Commence antibiotics (broad spectrum and
metronidazole)
(iii) IVI
a. Peripheral for fluid replacement
b. Central to monitor fluid replacement
(iv) Nasogastric tube
Aspirate gastric contents, as these patients are at grave
risk from aspiration
(v) Catheterise
To empty the bladder and subsequently monitor urine
output
3. Pre-incision
(i) General anaesthetic with endotracheal intubation
(ii) Position
Supine with a slight Trendelenberg tilt
(iii) Skin preparation of all abdomen and towel up for a left
paramedian incision
4. Incision
Lower left paramedian
5. Procedure
(i) Assess the problem
a. Obstructing carcinoma — Assess the degree of
obstruction and the tumour
(see general principle,
page 122)
b. Perforated diverticular disease — Mop out all faecal
contamination and
peform a full
peritoneal toilet
Sample for
microbiological
examination
c. Sigmoid volvulus — Reduce the volvulus
(ii) Mobilise the sigmoid colon (fibrous adhesions may
arise around either a tumour or diverticular disease)
(iii) Divide and ligate the branches of the inferior
mesenteric vessels to the sigmoid colon
(iv) Divide the peritoneal reflection from the sigmoid
mesentery as it descends around the upper third of the
rectum and mobilise the upper third of the rectum
(v) Beware damage to the left ureter
(vi) Place a soft bowel clamp across the lower descending
colon and a second soft bowel clamp across the upper
third of the rectum. Place crushing clamps 2 cm within
these on the bowel to be resected
(vii) Divide the sigmoid colon flush with the crushing
clamps and remove the specimen
(viii) Close the rectal stump in two layers

6. Closure
   (i) If these has been gross pelvic contamination then leave a corrugated drain to the pelvis after completion of the peritoneal lavage
   (ii) Bring the distal descending colon out through a 3 cm diameter circular incision lying midway between the anterior superior iliac spine and the umbilicus. Keep the soft bowel clamp in place until the abdomen is closed
   (iii) Close in layers
   (iv) Create the colostomy with 8–10 interrupted circumferential absorbable sutures
   (v) Place a colostomy bag over the stoma
7. Postoperative management
   (i) Commence oral fluid at the return of bowel sounds and solid food after the colostomy has passed faeces
   (ii) Remove the pelvic drain when drainage is minimal and the track has started to granulate (approx. 5 days)
   (iii) Investigations
       a. Histological examination of the specimen
       b. Microbiology results
   (iv) Subsequent reconnection of the descending colon to the rectal stump should be undertaken once the patient's condition has improved sufficiently to tolerate the procedure. The use of circular stapling gun for this has been described.
8. Complications
   (i) Those of colostomy (see transverse colostomy, page 120)
   (ii) Infection
       a. Pelvic abscess
       b. Wound infection
       c. Septicaemia

IVALON SPONGE REPAIR FOR COMPLETE RECTAL PROLAPSE

1. Indications
   Complete rectal prolapse (intussusception) in the elderly with no other pathological cause
2. Preoperative management
   (i) Investigations
       a. Barium enema/colonoscopy to exclude pathological cause for prolapse, especially intussusception of the rectum with a polyp/tumour
       b. Sigmoidoscopy
       c. Galvanic studies of the perineal musculature
       d. Urodynamic studies to assess bladder emptying
   (ii) Full bowel preparation (see principles of bowel preparation, page 116)

   (iii) Broad spectrum with metronidazole antibiotic
     prophylaxis
   (iv) IVI
   (v) Catheterise the bladder
3. Pre-incision
   (i) General anaesthetic with endotracheal intubation
   (ii) Position
     Supine
   (iii) Skin preparation of all of abdomen for a left
     paramedian incision
4. Incision
 Left paramedian
5. Procedure
   (i) Full laparotomy and pack the small bowel into the right
    hypochondrium
   (ii) Incise the peritoneum on both sides of the sigmoid
    mesocolon and continue down around the upper third
    of the rectum to mobilise the rectum and recto-sigmoid
    colon
   (iii) Divide the mesorectum posteriorly for the whole length
    of the rectum
   (iv) *Beware the presacral plexus*
   (v) Ligate and divide the lateral rectal ligaments containing
    the middle rectal vessels
   (vi) *Beware the ureters laterally*
   (vii) Mobilise the peritoneum anteriorly in the Pouch of
    Douglas as this forms the hernial sac which allows the
    prolapse to occur. Expose the vaginal vault
    musculature, the rectum is now fully mobilised
   (viii) Cut the piece of Ivalon sponge to conform with the
    normal anatomy and envelop the rectum (usually about
    20×10 cm)
   (ix) Suture the tail of the sponge to the presacral fascia at
    the level of the sacro-coccygeal junction with a nylon
    suture
   (x) Allow the rectum to fall back into the sacro-coccygeal
    curve and wrap the Ivalon around the rectum, suturing
    its four free corners to the anterior rectal muscle with
    single nylon sutures
   (xi) Suture the uppermost part of the mesorectum to the
    fascia overlying the lumbo sacral disc with a nylon
    suture
   (xii) Extraperitonealise the rectum by closing the pelvic
    peritoneum over it
6. Closure
   (i) No drains
   (ii) Close in layers

134 Aids to Operative Surgery

7. Postoperative management
    (i) Commence oral fluids at the return of bowel sounds and solids after the passage of faeces
    (ii) Long-term use of bulk laxatives or hydrophylic laxative may be necessary
    (iii) Perform regular rectal examinations in the postoperative period to prevent faecal impaction
8. Complications
    (i) Early
        a. Infection — Around the prosthesis as a result of foreign material implantation
                Wound infection (although the bowel is not opened)
        b. DVT — Pelvic surgery in an elderly patient (see principles of prevention, page 7)
        c. Faecal impaction
    (ii) Late
        a. Recurrent prolapse — < 10%
        b. Anal incontinence due to anal sphincter weakness may need a post-anal repair

PRINCIPLES OF HAEMORRHOID SURGERY

1. Management
    (i) Exclude predisposing anorectal pathology, especially carcinoma of the rectum
    (ii) Proctoscopy to examine the anal canal and haemorrhoids
    (iii) Sigmoidoscopy to examine the rectum
    (iv) Haemoglobin, as blood loss can be significant

A. First degree
No prolapse, but bleeding and discharge causes pruritis ani
Treat by submucosal injection of 5 ml of 5% phenol in almond oil immediately above the haemorrhoid and therefore above the dentate line (the limit of somatic sensation)

B. Second degree
    (i) Prolapse but withdraw spontaneously
    (ii) Treat by banding with tight rubber bands (Barron)
    (iii) Withdraw the haemorrhoid via the proctoscope with Barrons grasping forceps which have been passed through the band applicator
    (iv) Apply the band by releasing the band applicator over the base of the haemorrhoid, ensuring that this will be constricted above the dentate line

(v) Alternatives
    a. Lords manual dilatation of the anus ⎱ requires
    b. Cryosurgery   ⎰ general
                                                   anaesthetic

C. Third degree — Haemorrhoidectomy

1. Preoperative management
   Preparation — two disposable enemata, one the day before
   and one immediately prior to surgery
2. Pre-incision
   (i) General anaesthetic with endotracheal intubation
   (ii) Position
   Lithotomy
   (iii) Skin preparation of perineum and anal canal
   (iv) Surgeon sitting facing the perineum
3. Procedure
   (i) Insert Parkes anal speculum to display the haemorrhoid
   to be operated upon
   (ii) Grasp the haemorrhoid with a haemostatic forcep and
   retract towards the surgeon
   (iii) Incise the skin at the base of the haemorrhoid with
   scissors as a V-shaped incision
   (iv) Extend this incision into the mucosa either side of the
   haemorrhoid raising it off the muscles of the internal
   sphincter
   (v) Transfix and ligate the pedicle of the haemorrhoid with
   a silk suture leaving a long length of suture material
   attached. Excise the haemorrhoid 0.5 cm distal to the
   ligature
   (vi) Repeat the procedure with the other haemorrhoids
   (vii) *Leave a mucocutaneous bridge between each
   haemorrhoid to reduce any subsequent anal stricture*
   (viii) At the end place a small paraffin soaked pack to reduce
   bleeding within the anal canal, supported by a T-
   shaped bandage
4. Postoperative management
   (i) Encourage bowel action with adequate analgesia and
   bulk laxative
   (ii) Digital rectal examination at the fifth postoperative day
   to exclude anal stenosis and commence the daily use of
   an anal dilator
5. Complications
   (i) Early
   a. Haemorrhage — Reactionary
   b. Acute retention of urine
   c. Constipation with pain resulting in faecal impaction

      (ii) Late
          a. Anal stenosis
          b. Fissure
          c. Skin tags
          d. Recurrent haemorrhoids
          e. Incontinence with sphincter damage

TREATMENT OF ANAL FISSURE

Chronic anal fissures either lie posteriorly (90% in men, 60% in women) or anteriorly (10% in men, 40% in women) they must be differentiated from
      (i) Carcinoma of the anus
      (ii) Anal chancre
      (iii) TB
      (iv) herpes
          A careful search must be made for evidence of Crohn's disease, and less commonly, ulcerative colitis

A. **Manual dilatation of the anus**
    (Lord procedure)
    Contraindications
        (i) Patulous anus with mucosal prolapse
        (ii) Fibrous anal stricture
        (iii) Caution in the elderly since this may produce a complete rectal prolapse
    1. Preoperative management
       Rectal washout prior to surgery
    2. Pre-procedure
       (In the left lateral position)
           (i) General anaesthetic with an endotracheal tube as this procedure may induce laryngospasm
           (ii) Perform an examination under anaesthesia with a full sigmoidoscopy to exclude other pathology
    3. Procedure
           (i) Proceeding gently, insert the index and third fingers of each hand and dilate the internal sphincter laterally, relaxing and breaking down the spasm and fibrosis induced by the fissure
           (ii) Maintain for 3–4 minutes
           (iii) At the end place a small anal pack which is withdrawn once the patient is awake
    4. Postoperative management
           (i) Commence on a bulk laxative the next day and continue using a daily anal dilator for one month
           (ii) Complications
               a. Tearing (splitting of the anal canal)
               b. Mucosal prolapse
               c. Incontinence

B. Lateral sphincterotomy
 1. Preoperative management
    Rectal washout prior to surgery
 2. Pre-procedure
      (i) Either general or local anaesthetic (1% xylocaine with 1
           in 200,000 adrenaline) 5 ml into the base of the fissure
           and 5 ml at 3 o'clock on the anal verge
     (ii) Left lateral position
    (iii) Sigmoidoscopy to exclude coexisting pathology
 3. Procedure
      (i) Insert the left index finger into the anal canal
     (ii) Insert the blade of the sphincterotomy knife through the
           skin at the anal margin and pass it up in the
           subcutaneous tissue with the blade flat and parallel to
           the mucosa for 2–3 cm
    (iii) Rotate the cutting blade of the knife through 90° away
           from the lumen and divide the lower fibres of the
           internal sphincter. There will be a palpable 'give' when
           this is achieved
     (iv) Remove the knife and press to prevent haematoma
           formation
 4. Postoperatively
    Commence on a bulk laxative to soften the stool
 5. Complications
      (i) Incontinence if the external sphincter is also
           inadvertently divided
     (ii) Peri-anal haematoma
    (iii) Recurrent fissure

SURGERY FOR FISTULA IN ANO

A.   Pathological principles
 1. Goodsalls rule
      (i) All fistulae anterior to a coronal plane through the
           centre of the anus track radially to the recto-anal canal
     (ii) All fistulae posterior to this plane track circumferentially
           to enter the anorectal canal in the midline posteriorly
 2. Parkes' classification
      (i) *Low* (95%)
           a. Submucous/superficial
           b. Intersphincteric
           c. Transphincteric
     (ii) *High* (5%)
           a.   Suprasphincteric
           b.   Extrasphincteric

3. Simple versus complicated
    (i) Simple
        a. Direct track, not involving any sphincter, to the
           mucosa, although no internal opening is necessarily
           present
    (ii) Complicated
         Multiple peri-anal tracks or a high fistula
4. Exclude coexistent or causative pathology
    (i) Crohn's disease
    (ii) Carcinoma
    (iii) TB

B. Simple low fistulae
1. Preoperative management
   Rectal washout prior to surgery
2. Procedure
    (i) General anaesthetic
    (ii) Position
         Lithotomy
    (iii) Pass a probe from the fistula opening towards the anus;
          if there is no inner opening then push the probe
          through into the anal lumen
    (iv) Excise the fistula, leaving a wide gap between the
         skin/mucosa on each side to prevent 'bridging' resulting
         in a recurrent fistula
    (v) Send the specimen for histological examination
    (vi) Dress and support this with a T-bandage
3. Postoperative management
    (i) Daily bulk laxative and simple analgesia
    (ii) Histological examination of the specimen

C. Complicated/high fistula
    (i) Exclude underlying pathology (carcinoma and Crohn's
        disease)
    (ii) Consider defunctioning the anus with a transverse
         colostomy (see page 120) prior to definitive surgery
    (iii) Treatment is best undertaken in specialist centres and
          involves excision of the fistula track, defining the
          sphincter layers in the process and reconstruction of
          these layers as a primary or secondary procedure
    (iv) Alternatively, pass an absorbable suture (silk/nylon)
         through the length of the fistula and then tie the two
         ends together outside the anus. Gradually pull this
         through the layers encouraging fibrosis along its track
         and allowing drainage along the length of the suture
4. Complications
    (i) Recurrent fistulae and abscesses
    (ii) Faecal incontinence if a high fistula is treated
         inappropriately and the external sphincter is divided

PILONIDAL SINUS

1. Preoperative management
   (i) Carefully examine the natal cleft and locate all the openings both within the cleft and also laterally
   (ii) *Beware confusion with fistula in ano*
   Antibiotic prophylaxis is unnecessary
2. Pre-incision
   (i) Either general or local (xylocaine with adrenaline) anaesthetic
   (ii) Position
   Lateral or prone with buttocks abducted
   (iii) Skin preparation of natal cleft to anus and both buttocks
3. Procedure
   (i) Meticulously shave the region around the sinuses
   (ii) Gently probe and delineate all tracks
   (iii) Excise the midline pits in an elliptical incision
   (iv) Excise the lateral sinuses with a small circumference of surrounding skin
   (v) Curette out the sinus tracks
4. Closure
   (i) Either: regular dry dressings or silastic foam dressing and allow to granulate or
   (ii) Primary closure
5. Postoperative management
   Continue regular weekly shaving area adjacent to and including the sinus wound

PILONIDAL ABSCESS

   (i) Excise the roof as for pilonidal sinus
   (ii) Pus specimen for microbiological analysis
   (iii) Allow to granulate, avoid primary closure

Urology

URETHRAL CATHETERISATION

1. Objective
    (i) Diagnostic, therefore not self-retaining (short term, temporary or long term silastic intermittent self catheterisation)
    (ii) Therapeutic
        a. Urethral — Smallest self retaining
        b. (Suprapubic)
    (iii) Indications for a large bore catheter
        a. Clots
        b. Infected urine
2. Preparation
    (i) Position
        Supine
    (ii) Prepare the genitals with antiseptic, retracting the foreskin fully
    (iii) *Strict asepsis is essential*
    (iv) Local anaesthetic to urethra
    (v) Select catheter size
3. Procedure
    (i) Pass the appropriate catheter gently, without force
    (ii) Once in position
        a. Attach to a *closed* collecting system
        b. Inflate self retaining balloon
4. Complications
    (i) Unable to pass catheter: use either
        a. Narrower catheter
        b. Beaked Coude catheter
        c. Catheter introducer
        d. Suprapubic catheter
        e. Or seek assistance
    (ii) Significant haematuria
        Consider replacing with a larger 3-way irrigating catheter

URETHRAL DILATATION

1. Preoperative management
   (i) Investigations
      a. MSU
      b. Urethrogram
   (ii) Correct pre-existing urinary tract infection
   (iii) Empty the bladder immediately prior to the procedure
   (iv) Antibiotic cover is essential if there has been a recent urinary tract infection
   (v) Use either general or local (xylocaine gel) anaesthetic
2. Procedure
   (i) Position
      Supine
   (ii) *Strict asepsis essential*
   (iii) Meatal stricture
      a. Use either Hegar's dilator or female urethral dilator
      b. Start with the largest dilator which is passable with no resistence
      c. Never force the dilator
      d. Cease as soon as bleeding commences
   (iv) Urethral stricture
      Use either Cluttons or Liston's bougies
   (v) Notation on bougie
      Circumference at tip in mm (French gauge)
      Circumference of shaft in mm (French gauge)
   (vi) Always pass without force with the beak pointing dorsally on the penis
   (vii) Beware false passages
   (viii) Continue, using next larger size until the bougie is gripped; never force beyond this point
   (ix) Cease as soon as bleeding commences
3. Complications
   Failure to pass bougie
   a. Try a smaller size (< 14F use gum elastic bougie)
   b. If this fails, use filiforms (faggot method with a follower)
   c. Refer to a urologist for urethroplasty
4. Postoperative management
   MSU after procedure
5. Complications
   (i) False passage
   (ii) Urinary tract infection
      a. Ascending
      b. Septicaemia
   (iii) Stricture
      a. Recurrent
      b. Iatrogenic due to traumatic dilatation

CYSTOSCOPY, LITHOLOPAXY AND RETROGRADE URETEROGRAPHY

1. Preoperative management
   (i) Investigation
       a. MSU — correct UTI if present
       b. IVP
   (ii) Antibiotic cover if urine recently infected
2. Pre-procedure
   (i) Spinal, epidural or general anaesthetic (endotracheal tube if endoscopic resection anticipated)
   (ii) Position
        Lithotomy
   (iii) Skin preparation of all of external genitalia, retracting foreskin with a drape over the suprapubic area to allow palpation of the bladder

A. Cystoscopy
Procedure
   (i) Urethroscopy using a 30° telescope in the irrigating sheath down the urethra *with no force*
   (ii) Remove the obturator, empty the bladder, measuring the urine volume and collecting a specimen for microbiological examination
   (iv) Irrigate the bladder with isotonic saline solution, evacuate any clots or debris
   (v) Pass the 70° telescope with light source attached and visualise the distending bladder
   (vi) Examine the distended bladder, noting the air bubble, ureteric orifices, trigone and prostatic impression (Marion's sign)
   (vii) Remove the telescope, empty the bladder and replace the obturator prior to removal of the sheath
   (viii) Finish the procedure with a bimanual examination of the pelvis

B. Litholopaxy
1. Contraindications
   (i) Children < 10 years old
   (ii) Infected urine
   (iii) Urethral stricture
   (iv) Bladder pathology
        a. Diverticulum
        b. Carcinoma
        c. Tuberculosis
        d. Bilharzia

2. Needs
   (i) Antibiotic cover
   (ii) *General anaesthetic* with endotracheal intubation
3. Procedure
   (i) Pass the lithotrite, beak anteriorly into the bladder, insert a 30° telescope and fill the bladder with irrigating fluid.
   (ii) Visualise the stone and grasp it in the blades of the lithotrite
   (iii) Crush the stone into small fragments, withdraw the lithotrite, insert an irrigating sheath and irrigate the stone fragments for biochemical analysis

C. Retrograde ureterography

1. Indications
   (i) Delineation of the lower limit of a complete ureteric obstruction
   (ii) Pyelography in a poorly functioning kidney
2. Procedure
   (i) Pass the catheterising cystoscope and visualise the ureteric orifices and trigone
   (ii) Difficulty may arise in a very trabecullated bladder
   (iii) Gently pass a straight ureteric catheter (size 3F) up the ureter as far as the level to be visualised
   (iv) Withdraw the stillette and cystoscope, collect urine for cytological examination in suspected malignancy
   (v) Pyelography/ureterography by injection of Hypaque either in theatre using an image intensifier or transferring the patient to the x-ray department
   (vi) Remove ureteric catheter immediately after the procedure to reduce the risk of ascending infection
3. Postoperative management
   (i) MSU
   (ii) Litholopaxy: 3-way irrigating catheter
4. Complications
   (i) Infection
       a. Urinary tract
       b. Septicaemia
   (ii) Bladder perforation
       a. Intraperitoneal: laparotomy
       b. Extraperitoneal — Minor — Catheterise
                            Major   Laparotomy

   (iii) Urethral stricture
   (iv) Ureteric perforation

PRINCIPLES OF TRANSURETHRAL RESECTION OF PROSTATE (TURP)

1. Preoperative management
   - (i) Investigations
     - a. MSU — Treat existing urinary tract infection
     - b. IVP/ultrasound to assess residual urine volume and upper track dilatation
     - c. Tartrate labile acid phosphatase
     - d. Renal function
     - e. Urodynamic studies to show flow rate
   - (ii) IVI
   - (iii) Antibiotic prophylaxis for gram negative organisms
2. Pre-procedure
   - (i) Either general or epidural anaesthetic
   - (ii) Position
     Lithotomy
   - (iii) Prepare as for cystoscopy (see page 142)
3. Procedure
   - (i) Select a resectoscope sheath which will pass down the urethra without force
   - (ii) Problem: small meatus, perform meatotomy
   - (iii) Perform a cystoscopy and urethroscopy (see page 142) to exclude coexistent bladder pathology
   - (iv) Pass the resectoscope
   - (v) Irrigate with isotonic glycine (systemic entry of irrigation fluid will occur at the prostatic bed, isotonic solutions prevent red cell osmotic lysis, glycine equilbrates throughout the total body water and reduces the risk of cardiac overload)
   - (vi) Insert the resectoscope with a 30° telescope
   - (vii) Commence resection:
     - a. First — Circumferential resection of the bladder neck
     - b. Then resect the lateral lobes distally as far as the verumontanum
     - c. Never resect beyond the pink transverse fibres of the prostatic capsule or resect distal to the verumontanum
   - (viii) Coagulate all bleeding vessels as they arise
   - (ix) Using the irrigating resectoscope at intervals wash out the prostatic chipping from the bladder and send for histological examination
   - (x) At the end of the procedure, insert a three way irrigation catheter (22–24F) into the bladder and irrigate with glycine solution until the haematuria has subsided
4. Complications
   - (i) Early
     - a. Infection — Urine
       Septicaemia

  b. Bleeding — Reactionary
          Secondary   — Urinary infection
                         Carcinoma of the
                         prostate
  (ii) Late
     a. Recurrence of prostatism — Inadequate resection
                                   Urethral stricture
                                   Bladder neck stenosis
     b. Recurrent carcinoma
     c. Metastatic carcinoma
     d. Impotence
     e. Incontinence
     f. Retrograde ejaculation

RETROPUBIC PROSTATECTOMY

1. Preoperative management
   (i) Investigations as for TURP (see page 144)
   (ii) IVI
   (iii) Antibiotic prophylaxis to gram negative bacteria
2. Pre-incision
   (i) General anaesthetic with endotracheal intubation
   (ii) Position
      a. Initially lithotomy, perform cystoscopy to exclude
         coexistent bladder pathology
      b. Then supine with Trendelenberg tilt of 5° — Surgeon
         standing on the left side
   (iii) Skin preparation for a low abdominal incision with penis
         prepared and accessible
3. Incision
   Transverse suprapubic (Pfannenstial)
4. Procedure
   (i) Divide the linea alba and insert Millin's retractor to
       expose the cave of Retzius, depress the bladder with the
       third blade
   (ii) Place two small swabs, one each side in the lateral
        limits of the retropubic space
   (iii) Stay sutures to the prostatic capsule above and below
         the line of incision
   (iv) Incise the prostate capsule transversely 1–2 cm below
        the vesico prostatic junction. Control capsular bleeding
   (v) Divide the upper prostatic urethra with scissors and
       digitally enucleate the prostatic adenoma
   (vi) Remove the adenoma after division of the lower
        prostatic urethra
   (vii) Using Millin's bladder neck spreader visualise and
         excise the posterior overhanging bladder neck with any
         residual middle prostatic lobe

5. Closure
   (i) Pass an irrigating 3-way catheter per urethra into the
       bladder and inflate the balloon
   (ii) Close the anterior prostatic capsule with absorbable
        sutures
   (iii) Suction drain to the retropubic space
   (iv) Close in layers
   (v) During the closure irrigate the bladder with citrate
       solution to evacuate clots
6. Postoperative management
   As for TURP (see page 144) except: remove retropubic drain
   after urine has been successfully passed following removal
   of the catheter
7. Complications
   As for TURP (see page 144) — In addition
   Early
   a. DVT (pelvic surgery in the elderly)
   b. Osteitis pubis

APPROACH TO THE KIDNEY

A. **Anterior approach**
   Position
   Supine
1. Incision
   (i) Paramedian/Kochers subcostal on the appropriate side
   (ii) Full laparotomy
2. Procedure
   (i) Divide peritoneal reflection lateral to colon and mobilise
       the colonic flexure
   (ii) *Beware*
       a. *On right — Hepatic flexure*
                      Duodenum
                      Gonadal vessels
       b. *On left — Splenic flexure*
                     Spleen
                     Tail of pancreas
                     Gonadal vessels
   (ii) Mobilise the colon medially to display the perinephric
        fascia which is opened to display the kidney
   (iii) Structures at the hilum
        a. Renal vein is most anterior
        b. Renal artery
        c. Ureter is deep to the artery
   (iv) Postoperatively
        Ileus common

B. Posterior approach
Position lateral, with a renal bridge under the opposite loin
1. Incision
    (i) Either supracostal or subcostal, following the line of the 12th rib; commencing 6 cm lateral to the midline and finishing in the posterior axillary line
    (ii) Deepen by dividing
        a. Latissimus dorsi
        b. External oblique
        c. Internal oblique/quadratus lumborum in the line of the incision to display the perinephric fascia
        d. Identify the ureter
    (iii) Open the perinephric fascia to display the kidney
    (iv) Structures at the hilum
        a. Ureter is most posterior
        b. Renal artery
        c. Renal vein deep to the artery
    (v) *Beware pneumothorax*
    (vi) Ileus common with retroperitoneal trauma

NEPHRECTOMY

1. Indications
    (i) Malignant tumour arising within the kidney
    (ii) Chronic pyelonephritis complicated by hypertension, recurrent infection
    (iii) Transitional cell carcinoma of the ureter treated by nephro-ureterectomy,
2. Preoperative management
    (i) Examine and mark the side
    (ii) Investigations
        a. MSU and treat concurrent urinary tract infection
        b. IVP/ultrasound — Delineate pathology
                    Confirm the presence of opposite kidney
        c. Adenocarcinoma — Arteriography ± embolisation
                    Cavagram to exclude venous extension
        d. Transitional cell carcinoma — Cystoscopy to exclude bladder tumours
        e. Urine cytology
    (iii) Antibiotic prophylaxis to gram negative bacteria
    (iv) IVI
    (v) Catheterise
3. Pre-incision
    General anaesthetic with endotracheal intubation

4. Procedure
    (i) Use anterior approach (see page 146) but do not open perinephric fascia when operating for cancer
    (ii) Clamp the renal artery
    (iii) Ligate and divide in continuity
        a. Renal vein (oversew the short right renal vein)
        b. Renal artery
    (iv) Adenocarcinoma of the kidney/chronic pyelonephritis
        Ligate and divide ureter at an accessible point. Remove kidney for histological examination
    (v) Transitional cell carcinoma of the renal pelvis
        Needs a complete ureterectomy with excision of the vesico ureteric junction and formal closure of the bladder

5. Closure
    (i) Large suction drain to the renal bed
    (ii) Close in layers

6. Postoperative management
Investigation
    a. MSU
    b. Histological examination of specimen
    c. Transitional cell carcinoma — Needs long-term cystoscopic follow-up

7. Complications
    (i) Early
        a. Infection — Urine
                       Wound
                       Septicaemia
        b. Haemorrhage — Reactionary at renal pedicle
        c. Ileus
        d. DVT
    (ii) Late
        Tumour recurrence, new primary with transitional cell carcinoma

PYELOLITHOTOMY/URETEROLITHOTOMY

1. Preoperative management
    (i) Examine and mark the side
    (ii) Investigations
        a. MSU, treat pre-existing urinary tract infection
        b. IVP
        c. Those for renal calculi (24 h urine for calcium, oxalate, urate, xanthine, cysteine analysis)
        d. Renal function (electrolytes, clearance studies)
        e. Plain abdominal x-ray en route to the operating theatre to see if the stone has moved

    (iii) Broad spectrum antibiotic prophylaxis
    (iv) IVI
2. Pre-incision
    (i) General anaesthetic with endotracheal intubation
    (ii) Position
        Lateral for pyelolithotomy, supine for ureterolithotomy

A. Pyelolithotomy
(Stone in pelvis/upper ureter)
1. Incision
   posterior approach (see page 147)
2. Procedure
    (i) Assess and gently mobilise the kidney (beware perinephric inflammation and fibrosis)
    (ii) Controlling the stone with the left hand retract the renal sinus with a GilVernet retractor
    (iii) Incise the renal pelvis over the stone in its long axis and remove the stone with Desjardins forceps. Wash out pelvis
    (iv) on table pyelogram
    (v) Close the renal pelvis with interrupted absorbable sutures
    (vi) Send the stone for biochemical analysis
3. Closure
    (i) Drains
       a. One to the renal pelvis
       b. One to the wound
    (ii) Close in layers

B. Ureterolithotomy
(Stones in middle third of ureter)
1. Incision
    (i) Extended grid iron in iliac fossa
    (ii) Do not open peritoneum
2. Procedure
    (i) Sweep the peritoneum medially and locate the ureter
    (ii) Place slings around the ureter above and below the stone
    (iii) Gently milk the stone proximally as there may be ulceration/fibrosis of the ureter where it has impacted
    (iv) Incise onto the stone and remove it for biochemical analysis
    (v) Pass a ureteric catheter distally to exclude distal obstruction
    (vi) Close the ureter with absorbable suture
3. Closure
    (i) Drain the retroperitoneal space
    (ii) Close in layers

4. Postoperative management
   (i) Remove the drain when drainage is minimal
   (ii) Investigations
      a. Biochemical analysis of stones
      b. MSU
5. Complications
   (i) Early
      a. Infection — Urine
                     Septicaemia
      b. Stone fragmented during removal — Small (< 1 cm)
                                           fragments should
                                           pass
                                           spontaneously
                                           Larger
                                           irretrievable
                                           fragments, refer
                                           to specialist
                                           centre
      c. Hydronephrosis — Ureteric oedema
                          Residual calculous obstruction
   (ii) Late
      a. Recurrent calculi
      b. Hydronephrosis — Ureteric stricture
                          Recurrent calculi

PRINCIPLES OF PYELOPLASTY

1. Indications
   Idiopathic pelvi ureteric junction (PUJ) obstruction
2. Preoperative management
   (i) Examine and mark the side
   (ii) Investigations
      a. MSU
      b. IVP
      c. Isotope renogram to assess the effect of the
         obstruction on renal function
   (iii) Antibiotic prophylaxis for gram negative bacteria
   (iv) IVI
3. Procedure
   (i) General anaesthetic with endotracheal intubation
   (ii) Use posterior approach to the kidney (see page 147)
   (iii) Needs a full exposure of the kidney and pelvis
   (iv) Type of pyeloplasty depends on the size of the renal
        pelvis
   (v) *Large baggy pelvis*: *Anderson-Hynes pyeloplasty*
      a. Divide the ureter just below the PUJ
      b. Excise the baggy redundant renal pelvis 1–2 cm from
         and parallel to the renal sinus

c. Close the upper two-thirds of the renal pelvis with an absorbable continuous suture
d. Incise the opened end of the upper ureter longitudinally on its lateral side to match the size of the opening in the lower third of the renal pelvis
e. Pass a nephrostomy tube through the anastomosis
f. Anastomose the upper ureter to the lower third of the renal pelvis

(vi) *Moderate pelvis*: *Culp pyeloplasty*
a. Make a 6 cm longitudinal incision equidistant either side of the PUJ
b. At the top of this incision curve it round medially and then continue it back down to the PUJ, 1 cm medial and parallel to the first incision to fashion a pedicled flap based on the PUJ
c. Rotate this flap through 180° to point inferiorly and suture onto the lower part of the incision below the PUJ with continuous absorbable sutures
d. Close the defect in the PUJ from where the flap originated with continuous absorbable sutures

(vii) *Small pelvis*: *Foley pyeloplasty*
a. Make a Y shaped incision with the lower vertical arm commencing just above the PUJ and extending for 2 cm beyond it down the ureter
b. Convert it to a V shaped incision (Y-V plasty) and close with a continuous absorbable suture

4. Closure
   (i) Splint the pyeloplasty with a Malecot catheter brought out as a nephrostomy
   (ii) Suction drain to the renal bed
   (iii) Close in layers, draining the wound

5. Postoperative management
   (i) Remove the drain when dry
   (ii) Remove the nephrostomy tube 10 days postoperatively
   (iii) Investigate
       a. MSU
       b. IVP to assess pyeloplasty

6. Complications
   (i) Infection
       a. Urine
       b. Wound
       c. Septicaemia
   (ii) Pyeloplasty leakage
       a. Usually close spontaneously
   (iii) Recurrent obstruction
       a. Usually oedema
       b. Rarely, recurrent PUJ obstruction or fibrosis

PRINCIPLES OF RENAL TRANSPLANTATION

1. Donors — 20% live related
   (i) From immediate family
      a. Non diabetic
      b. Healthy and normotensive
      c. Two normal kidneys — IVP
                                 Arteriogram
      d. No concurrent infection
      e. No hereditary renal disorders (e.g. polycystic disease)
   (ii) Remove kidney by either anterior or posterior approach
        with great care to the pedicle, preserving as much
        ureter as possible with the kidney
2. Donors — 80% cadaveric
   (i) Brain stem death
      a. Trauma — 25%
      b. CVA — 40%
      c. Other cause — 35%
   (ii) Contraindications
      a. >70 years of age
      b. Hypertensive
      c. Diabetes
      d. Systemic infection
      e. Extra-cranial malignant tumour
      f. Renal disease
   (iii) Problems
      a. Diagnostic criteria for brain death
      b. Consent from relatives and coroner (UK), donor card
         consent
      c. Must be fully ventillated prior to removal of organs
   (iv) Use abdominal approach
      a. Allows removal of both kidneys *en bloc* with cava
         and aorta
      b. Allows removal of other organs (liver, pancreas)
3. Recipient
   (i) Compatability
      a. HLA
      b. ABO
      c. Mixed lymphocyte culture
   (ii) Investigations
      a. Gastroscopy — Coexisting peptic ulcer
      b. MSU and treat urinary tract infection
   (iii) Correct
      a. Hypertension
      b. Secondary hyperparathyroidism
      c. Osteomalacia
      d. Hypersplenism

    (iv) Consider recipient nephrectomy
       a. Hypertensive chronic renal failure
       b. Polycystic disease, to make room
       c. Chronic pyelonephritis
4. Transplant operation
    (i) Cold kidney time — Up to 72 hours
    (ii) General anaesthesia with endotracheal intubation
5. Incision
   Extended grid iron (Rutherford Morrison) in the opposite iliac fossa to the donor side
6. Procedure
    (i) Place donor kidney extra peritoneally
    (ii) Anastomose
       a. Renal artery to internal iliac artery end-to-end
       b. (20% have double artery so use a cuff of aorta for anastomosis to external iliac artery)
       c. Renal vein to external iliac vein end-to-side
       d. Ureter to bladder
6. Postoperative management
    (i) Immunosuppression
       a. Azothioprine
       b. Cortico steroids
       c. Anti lymphocyte globulin
       d. Cyclosporin
    (ii) Monitor
       a. Urine output and osmolality (encourage diuresis to diminish the chances of acute tubular necrosis)
       b. ECG
       c. Serum potassium
       d. CVP
       e. *Beware wound haematoma*
7. Complications
    (i) Early
       a. Oliguria/anuria — Radioisotope renogram
                         IVP
                         Renal angiography
                         Biopsy graft
       b. Renal artery stenosis/leakage
       c. Ureteric stenosis/leakage
       d. Infection — Urine   ⎫ Viral
                  Wound ⎬ Fungal
                  Graft   ⎭ Protozoal
                  Septicaemia
    (ii) Late
       a. Immunosuppression — Opportunistic infection
                                   Lymphoma
       b. Tertiary hyperparathyroidism

8. Rejection
    (i) Hyperacute
        a. Within hours
        b. Due to platelet occlusion as a result of prior sensitisation
   (ii) *Acute*
        a. Up to 6 months
        b. Cell mediated
  (iii) *Chronic*
        a. 12–18 months
        b. Occlusion due to arteriolar intimal thickening
9. Assessment of rejection
    (i) Clinically
        a. Tender graft
        b. Malaise with pyrexia
   (ii) Decreased renal function
        a. Decreased output
        b. Acute renal failure with rising creatinine (>10% change is significant)
  (iii) *Isotope renogram*
   (iv) *Percutaneous biopsy/aspiration cytology*
10. Results
    (i) Operative mortality — 4%
        a. Infection
        b. GI haemorrhage
        c. CVA
        d. Myocardial infarction
   (ii) *Graft survival*

	1 year	5 years
Related donor	90%	80%
Cadaveric donor	80%	60%

PRINCIPLES OF URINARY DIVERSION

1. Classify
    (i) Temporary
   (ii) Permanent
2. Indications
    (i) Distal obstruction
   (ii) Incurable fistula
  (iii) Cystectomy
   (iv) Loss of external sphincter
    (v) Ectopia vesicae
   (vi) Calculi

3. Problems with diversion
    (i) Urine collection
   (ii) Ascending urinary infection
  (iii) Reflux
  (iv) Anastomotic stricture
   (v) Solute reabsorbtion
  (vi) Carcinogenic effect of solutes

Methods
1. Nephrostomy
    (i) Temporary ⎱ Use a Malecot open
   (ii) Permanent ⎰ percutaneous catheter
2. Pyelostomy
    (i) Catheter
   (ii) Loop
3. Ureterostomy
      Temporary catheterisation
    (i) From above
   (ii) Retrograde
      Permanent
    (i) Unilateral ureteric disease
        a. High pathology — Uretero-ureterostomy
                            Ileal loop interposition
                            Autotransplant kidney to iliac
                            fossa
        b. Low pathology — Ureteric bladder
                           reimplantation
                           Boari flap
                           Psoas bladder hitch
   (ii) bilateral (following cystectomy)
        a. Uretero cutaneous anastomosis (high incidence of
           stomal stricture)
        b. Ileal conduit
        c. Colonic implantation (ascending infection,
           hyperchloraemic acidosis and increased incidence of
           carcinoma of the distal colon)
        d. Lowsley's operation (rectal bladder)
      Bladder
    (i) Suprapubic catheterisation
   (ii) Urethral catheterisation
  (iii) Urethrotomy

CYSTECTOMY AND ILEAL CONDUIT

1. Plan of treatment for transitional carcinoma of the bladder
    (i) T_1 carcinoma
        a. Endoscopic resection — Review

     b. Multiple recurrent tumours; consider intra vesical
        chemotherapy (adriomycin, mitomycin, thiotepa,
        epodyl)
  (ii) T_2 carcinoma
     Endoscopic resection — Review, if recurs as T_2 then
     proceed to radiotherapy as for T_3
  (iii) T_3 carcinoma
     a. 5,500 CGy radiotherapy to the tumour in fractions
        then either
     b. Review, if recurs then cystectomy
     c. Proceed to cystectomy at completion of radiotherapy
  (iv) T_4 carcinoma
     5,500 CGy radiotherapy to palliate symptoms with
     urinary diversion ± cystectomy
2. Preoperative management
   (i) Examine the patient standing, sitting and lying flat to
       find a suitable point in the right iliac fossa to site the
       ileal conduit
   (ii) Investigations
       a. IVP
       b. Cystoscopy with biopsy and bimanual examination
       c. Pelvic CT scan/pelvic ultrasound
       d. Pelvic lymphangiogram
       e. Distant metastases — Chest X-ray
                                Liver ultrasound/isotope scan
                                Skeletal survey/isotope bone
                                scan
   (iii) Antibiotics — broad spectrum with metronidazole
                       prophylaxis
   (iv) Bowel preparation (see page 116)
   (v) IVI
   (vi) Nasogastric tube
3. Pre-incision
   (i) General anaesthesia with endotracheal intubation
   (ii) Position
       Supine with steep Trendelenberg tilt
   (iii) Skin preparation of all of abdomen and external
         genitalia, including vagina
4. Incision
   Left lower paramedian commencing just above symphysis
5. Procedure
   (i) Full laparotomy
       a. Exclude intra-abdominal metastases
       b. Assess tumour fixity
   (ii) Expose and dissect out each ureter from the level of
        the bifurcation of the common iliac arteries downwards,
        divide the ureters at this level ligating the distal ends,
        mobilising the proximal ends

   (iii) Ligate both internal iliac arteries in continuity (except in arteriopaths when this may compromise the leg circulation)

   (iv) Mobilise the bladder from the symphysis by blunt dissection of the retropubic space

   (v) Laterally
   a. Divide the vas in the male
   b. Mobilise and divide the ovarian and uterine pedicles in the female
   c. Clamp, divide and ligate the vesical pedicles containing the superior and inferior vesical vessels

   (vi) *Male*
   a. Bluntly dissect down around the prostate to separate the urethra and rectum
   b. Lifting the bladder and prostate upwards, clamp and divide the urethra
   c. Peel the prostate and vesicles off the rectum, divide the lateral peritoneal attachment of the bladder and remove the specimen

   (vii) *Female*
   a. Bluntly dissect the retropubic space, lifting the bladder to palpate the urethra. Divide the urethra as distally as possible
   b. Open the inferior anterior wall of the vagina transversely and divide each lateral wall up to the cervix
   c. Divide the lateral vesical and uterine attachments to deliver the bladder, uterus, ovaries and anterior wall of the vagina *en bloc*
   d. Close the vagina

   (viii) Dissect out all the pelvic lymph nodes bilaterally for histology
   a. Obturator nodes
   b. Internal iliac chain
   c. Common iliac chain

   (ix) Pack the pelvis to reduce bleeding during the fashioning of the ileal conduit

6. Ileal conduit
   (i) Select a loop of distal ileum 20 cm in length commencing about 50 cm from the ileocaecal junction

   (ii) Isolate this loop and anastomose the two ends of the bowel with the loop lying below the mesentery

   (iii) Carefully mobilise the mesentery, avoid damage to the vascular arcades supplying both the loop and the remaining bowel

   (iv) Slit the distal free ends of the ureters for 2 cm and anastomose the splayed ends in a single layer of absorbable suture

    (v) Pass ureteric catheters up each ureter and into the
       proximal end of the ileal loop. Pass these catheters the
       whole length of the conduit
   (vi) Anastomose the ureters to the proximal end of the ileal
       conduit in a single layer of absorbable suture
  (vii) Complete the conduit by bringing out the distal ileal
       loop as a spout at the predetermined site in the right
       iliac fossa

7. Closure
    (i) Withdraw the pelvic pack and replace with a Foley
       balloon catheter passed per urethra, haemostasis is
       assisted by the balloon being fully inflated and placed
       on traction
   (ii) Drain the pelvis
  (iii) Close in layers

8. Postoperative management
    (i) Remove
       a. Pelvic urethral catheter at 24–48 hours
       b. Pelvic drain when drainage is minimal
       c. Ureteric catheters at 4–5 days
   (ii) Investigations
      Histological examination of specimen and pelvic lymph
      nodes

9. Complications
    (i) Early
       a. Haemorrhage from pelvic veins
       b. Rectal perforation (should be repaired and
         defunctioning colostomy)
       c. Infection — Urinary tract
                   Pelvic abscess
                   Septicaemia
       d. Ileus/obstruction with adhesions
   (ii) Late
       a. Stricture at uretero-ileal anastomosis
       b. Tumour recurrence
       c. Strangulation of ileal conduit — Volvulus
                                  Prolapse

10. Prognostic factors
    (i) Stage of tumour (TNM)
   (ii) Histological grade
  (iii) Tumour size

11. Prognosis
    5 years' survival
        a. T_1 — > 70%
        b. T_2 — 50%
        c. T_3 — 20%
        d. T_4 — 0%

CIRCUMCISION

1. Indications
    (i) Religious/social
    (ii) Phimosis
    (iii) Recurrent balanitis (especially diabetics)
    (iv) Prelude to radiotherapy for carcinoma of the penis
2. Pre-incision
    (i) General anaesthetic, optional caudal block reduces postoperative pain
    (ii) Position
       Supine
    (iii) Skin preparation of all of external genitalia, in childhood phimosis gently break down the preputial adhesions with a probe, retract the foreskin and clean the glans
3. Procedure
    (i) Apply two straight artery forceps side by side along the midline of the dorsum of the foreskin
    (ii) Incise between these two forceps with scissors to within 0.5 cm of the corona
    (iii) Continue this incision circumferentially around the foreskin in both directions. Pick up any bleeding vessels in artery forceps
    (iv) *Beware retraction of bleeding vessels*
    (v) *Do not use diathermy on the penis*
    (vi) The two incisions meet at the frenulum; place a clip across this and excise the foreskin distal to this
    (vii) Transfix the frenulum with an absorbable suture
    (viii) Ligate the vessels with absorbable sutures
    (ix) Suture the two layers of the foreskin with several interrupted absorbable sutures
    (x) Dress loosely
4. Complications
    (i) Infants may go into retention with pain
    (ii) After dissection of extensive prepucial adhesions, there may be considerable ulceration of the glans which may result in meatal stenosis

DARTOS POUCH ORCHIDOPEXY FOR UNDESCENDED/ECTOPIC TESTIS

1. Reasons for surgery
    (i) 90% have associated inguinal hernia
    (ii) May improve spermatogenesis
    (iii) Reduces risk of torsion (which is greater for undescended and ectopic testes)

(iv) Cosmetic/psychological
(v) Does *not* reduce the increased risk of malignant change in the testis but does render such change more immediately obvious to the patient
(vi) Optimal time to operate
Before 2 years old
(vii) If impalpable
Localise with ultrasound
(viii) If bilateral
Exclude anorchism by measuring the serum testosterone response to an injection of HCG (no response = anorchic)
2. Preoperative management
Examine the patient
a. Exclude retractile testis
b. Mark the side
3. Pre-incision
(i) General anaesthetic
(ii) Position
Supine
(iii) Skin preparation of all of genitalia and groin on relevant side
4. Incision
Groin skin crease
5. Procedure
(i) Open inguinal canal by dividing external oblique aponeuris from the external ring and locate the testes
a. 90% of undescended testes lie within the inguinal canal
b. 80% of ectopic testes lie in the superficial inguinal pouch
(ii) Carefully open the layers of the cord and dissect out the indirect inguinal hernia
(iii) Perform a herniotomy (see inguinal hernia repair, page 13)
(iv) Gently separate all the fibres of cremaster from the components of the cord until the vas and vessels lie free, thus lengthening these structures without tension
(v) Dartos pouch
a. Insert the left index finger into the scrotum from above
b. Make a 1 cm incision into the skin of the scrotum and pass artery forceps through the dartos layer up to the groin, grasp the mobilised testis and bring down to lie between the dartos and skin of the scrotum
6. Closure
(i) No drains
(ii) Close in layers

7. Postoperative management
   Most children can go home the same evening
8. Complications
   - (i) Small atrophic testis at operation
     Excise
   - (ii) Failed reduction
     Gain as much length with the first operation then subsequently re-explore and mobilise into scrotum
   - (iii) Early
     Testicular infarction with cord damage
   - (iv) Late
     Malignant change ($\times$ 20–30 incidence of malignancy of normal testis)
   - (v) If reduction fails or the testis lost, the optimal age for a testicular prosthesis implant is 15 years

HYDROCELE: LORDS OPERATION

1. Preoperative management
   - (i) Children
     Manage as inguinal hernia (see page 13)
   - (ii) Adult
     a. Careful history and examination; mark the side
     b. Exclude — Testicular tumour
     Trauma
     Epididymoorchitis
     c. If bilateral — Exclude ascites
     d. Aspirate
     Culture
     Cytology
     Always examine testis after aspiration
2. Pre-incision
   - (i) General or local anaesthetic
   - (ii) Position
     Supine
   - (iii) Skin preparation of all of external genitalia
3. Incision
   Transversely across the hemiscrotum through all layers including the hydrocele sac
4. Procedure
   - (i) Control bleeding from cut edges and suck out hydrocele fluid
   - (ii) Place 3 interrupted sutures each side of the testis, commencing at the edge of the sac, picking up several bites of the sac and finishing on the tunica at the junction of testis and epididymis
   - (iii) When all 6 sutures are in place, tighten them up to plicate the sac, obliterating the hydrocele and tie them

    (iv) Ensure absolute haemostasis
     (v) No drains
    (vi) Close in layers
  5. Postoperative management
     Apply a scrotal support for comfort
  6. Complications
     Scrotal haematoma

EXCISION OF VARICOCELE

  1. Preoperative management
     (i) Investigations
        a. If for infertility — Sperm count and analysis
        b. IVP for left sided varicocele has a pick up rate for
           renal carcinoma of < 1%
     (ii) Examine and mark the side with the patient standing
  2. Pre-incision
     (i) General anaesthetic
     (ii) Position
        Supine
     (iii) Skin preparation of groin
  3. Incision
     Groin skin crease
  4. Procedure
     (i) Open inguinal canal by dividing external oblique
         aponeurosis from the external ring
     (ii) Open the layers of the cord to display the distended
          pampiniform plexus/testicular vein branches
     (iii) Dissect out all the pampiniform plexus, ligate and divide
           all these veins
  5. Closure
     (i) Meticulous haemostasis
     (ii) No drains
     (iii) Close in layers
  6. Postoperative management
     Investigations — Infertility — Testicular biopsy
     Serial sperm analyses
  7. Complications
     (i) Early
        a. Scrotal haemotoma
        b. Damage to cord — Vas
                              Vessels
     (ii) Late
        Recurrent varicocele

ORCHIDECTOMY FOR TESTICULAR TUMOUR

  1. Preoperative management
     (i) Informed consent for orchidectomy, examine and mark
         the side

     (ii) Consider pre-treatment sperm banking
   (iii) Investigations
       a. Ultrasound — Primary tumour
                   Para-aortic nodes
                   Liver (with liver isotope scan)
       b. Chest X-ray
       c. Lymphangiography of para-aortic nodes
       d. Isotope bone scan
       e. Abdominal and thoracic CT
       f. 24 hour urine β-HCG — 80% of teratomas show elevation, especially malignant teratoma trophoblastic 5% of seminomas show elevation
       g. Blood — α-Feto protein elevated in teratoma
2. Pre-incision
     (i) General anaesthetic
    (ii) Position
       Supine
   (iii) Skin preparation of groin region
3. Incision
   Groin skin crease
4. Procedure
     (i) Open the inguinal canal by dividing the external oblique aponeurosis commencing from the external ring
    (ii) Mobilise the cord within the canal and cross clamp it
   (iii) Divide the cord and ligate the two ends with non-absorbable ligatures
   (iv) Deliver the testis by traction to the distal cord, thus inverting the scrotum, ligate and divide the gubernaculum
    (v) Send the specimen for histological examination
5. Closure
     (i) No drains
    (ii) Close in layers
6. Postoperative management
     (i) Apply a scrotal support for comfort
    (ii) Investigations
       a. Histological examination of the tumour
       b. Serial investigations for tumour markers since metastases may now become biochemically apparent
7. Complications
   Scrotal haematoma

Orthopaedic surgery

PRINCIPLES OF SURGERY FOR RHEUMATOID ARTHRITIS

1. Types of surgery
   - (i) Early rheumatoid synovectomy
     - a. Large joints
     - b. Metacarpo phalangeal joints
   - (ii) Intermediate rheumatoid
     - a. Divide synovial adhesions
     - b. Repair tendons
   - (iii) Advanced rheumatoid
     - a. Arthrodesis
     - b. Arthroplasty — Excision
       - Hemi
       - Surface
       - Total
2. Preoperative management
   - (i) If on steroids, then increase for the duration of the operation and immediate postoperative period
   - (ii) Broad spectrum antibiotic cover
   - (iii) *Beware rheumatoid involving cervical spine resulting in instability*
     Therefore
     - a. Cervical spine X-rays
     - b. Support the neck with a cervical collar during the anaesthetic
     - c. Consider fixation of the cervical spine
3. Principles of surgery
   - (i) The aim of surgery is to reduce pain and restore joint function
   - (ii) Use straight incisions
   - (iii) Delicate tissues must be handled carefully

Specific sites
 1. Shoulder
     (i) Avoid arthrodesis (since further incapacitates the
         polyarthritic and the bone is often softened)
    (ii) Consider — Synovectomy
                   — Total shoulder replacement (Kessel or
                     Stanmore)
 2. Elbow
     (i) Synovectomy
    (ii) Excision arthroplasty of the head of the radius
   (iii) Ulnar nerve decompression and transposition (see page
         167)
    (iv) Excise rheumatoid nodules
     (v) Total joint replacement if pain very severe
 3. Hand
     (i) Carpal tunnel — Release (see page 162)
    (ii) Trigger finger — Release (excise synovium)
   (iii) Rupture
         a. Repair or reimplant insertion
         b. Tendon transfer (e.g. extensor indicis to extensor
            pollicis longus)
    (iv) Tendons — Tenosynovitis — Tenolysis
     (v) Joints
         a. MCP — Early — Synovectomy
                  Late—Arthroplasty— Excise MC heads
                                     Total: Swanson
                                     silastic
         b. Thereby correcting — Ulnar drift
                                 dropped heads
         c. PIP — synovectomy — Reduces pain and swelling
                                Does *not* improve function
         d. Boutonniere deformity — Early — Operate
                                    Late — Leave
         e. Swan neck deformity —Arthrodesis   ⎫
                                                     ⎬ Equal
                        Swanson arthroplasty⎭ results

         f. DIP — Leave
 4. Thumb
     (i) Ulnar collateral ligament laxity
         Arthroplasty
    (ii) Carpo metacarpal joint
         a. Arthrodesis
         b. Trapezium replacement (Swanson silastic) equally
            effective
   (iii) *Beware carpal silastic implant dislocation*
    (iv) Therefore, plaster of Paris for 6 weeks
 5. Hip
    Total hip replacement (see page 174)

6. Knee
  (i) Early
    a. Synovectomy
    b. Excise popliteal cyst
  (ii) Late
    a. Arthroplasty — Surface
                      Hinge
                      Semi constrained
    b. Avoid arthrodesis in softened bone
    c. Causes undue stress on other joints

PUTTI PLATT OPERATION FOR RECURRENT DISLOCATION OF THE SHOULDER

1. Preoperative management
  (i) Confirm diagnosis by apprehension test — Abduction with external rotation
  (ii) Mark the side
  (iii) Check the axillary nerve is intact
  (iv) Investigations
       X-rays
    a. AP and lateral in abduction
    b. Arthrogram
2. Pre-incision
  (i) General anaesthetic with endotracheal intubation
  (ii) Position
       Supine
  (iii) Skin preparation of neck to lower chest, axilla, shoulder, arm to elbow
  (iv) Towel up arm separately with shoulder exposed
3. Incision
   Medial border of anterior deltoid to clavicle, then posteriorly to acromion
4. Procedure
  (i) Access to joint
    a. Reflect skin flap laterally and retract medially or divide cephalic vein
    b. Explore the delto pectoral cleft
    c. Divide acromial branch of acromio thoracic artery between ligatures
    d. Divide proximal deltoid 1 cm from its origin medial to lateral for the width of the incision
    e. Retract medially — Coracobrachialis
                          Short head of biceps thereby exposing subscapularis and its tendon, which is divided 1 cm from its insertion

(ii) Once the joint is opened, inspect
  a. Inside of the capsule
  b. Head of humerus
  c. Glenoid
  d. Place the arm in 15° of flexion and 90° of internal rotation, suture the lateral cuff of subscapularis to the anterior aspect of the glenoid with interrupted non-absorbable sutures

5. Closure
  (i) Suture medial subscapularis to its lateral tendon superficially
  (ii) Drain — suction deep to deltoid
  (iii) Repair deltoid
  (iv) Skin

6. Postoperative care
  (i) Keep arm in internal rotation with a sling to support the elbow for 6 weeks
  (ii) Use hand immediately
  (iii) Check position with X-ray

ULNAR NERVE TRANSPOSITION

1. Indications: ulnar nerve symptoms
  (i) Following fracture of either condyle of the humerus
  (ii) Osteoarthritis resulting in osteophytes at the elbow
  (iii) Recurrent dislocation of the nerve
  (iv) Excessive carrying angle
  (v) Idiopathic

2. Preoperative management
  (i) Examine, mark the side and fully document any neurological deficit (sensory deficit in little, ring finger; weakness of interossi with adduction/abduction of fingers)
  (ii) Investigations
    a. PA and lateral X-rays of elbow
    b. EMG studies of ulnar nerve
    c. Sickle test prior to tourniquet in negroes

3. Pre-incision
  (i) General anaesthetic
  (ii) Exsanguinate the arm and apply an arm tourniquet at 250 mmHg, *note the time*
  (iii) Position
    Supine with the arm extended and abducted on a side table
  (iv) Skin preparation of upper arm to wrist

4. Incision
  10 cm incision following the ulnar nerve and centred on the medial epicondyle

5. Procedure
    (i) Expose and mobilise the nerve, carefully preserving its blood supply
    (ii) Incise flexor carpi ulnaris between its two heads. Divide the medial intermuscular septum to expose the nerve
    (iii) *Beware: motor branch to flexor carpi ulnaris*
    (iv) Separate the common flexor origin from the medial epicondyle and place the nerve anterior to the medial epicondyle
6. Closure
    (i) Secure the nerve with interrupted absorbable sutures in the overlying soft tissues
    (ii) Suction drain to the wound
    (iii) Close the skin and apply a firm dressing
    (iv) Release the tourniquet, documenting the tourniquet time
7. Postoperative management
    Encourage early mobilisation
8. Complications
    (i) Ulnar nerve neuropraxia should recover quickly
    (ii) Damage motor branch to flexor carpi ulnaris

CARPAL TUNNEL OPERATION

1. Preoperative management
    (i) Examine the patient and mark the side, note any neurological deficit, especially to muscles of the thenar eminence
    (ii) Investigations
        a. Exclude aetiological factors — Rheumatoid
                                Diabetes
        b. Diagnostic — EMG studies of median nerve function
        c. Sickle status in negroes prior to tourniquet
2. Pre-incision
    (i) General anaesthetic with exsanguination of the arm or Biers block
    (ii) Exsanguinate the arm and inflate an arm tourniquet to 250 mmHg.
    (iii) *Note the time*
    (iv) Position
        Supine with arm extended on a side table
    (v) Skin preparation of all of hand and forearm, towel up with hand exposed and extended (assisted by a 'lead hand')
3. Incision
    Commencing at distal flexor crease of wrist and extending for 6 cm, 1 cm medial to thenar crease
4. Procedure
    (i) Deepen through deep forearm fascia proximally and palmar fascia distally

(ii) In this medial position the incision should avoid
   a. *Proximally — Superficial branch of median nerve*
   b. *Distally — Recurrent motor branch of medial nerve to the thenar eminence*
(iii) Visualise the median nerve proximal to the flexor retinaculum lying on the tendons of flexor digitorum sublimis
(iv) Insert a Macdonald dissector under the proximal border of the flexor retinaculum to protect the median nerve and divide the retinacular fibres longitudinally with a scalpel
(v) Direct the division to the ulnar side at its distal end to avoid the recurrent motor branch of the nerve. Divide all the fibres of the retinaculum
(vi) Gently retract the nerve and flexor tendons to inspect the underlying flexor surface of the carpus for ganglia which should be excised

5. Closure
  (i) Close the skin and apply a pressure dressing
  (ii) Release the tourniquet and document the tourniquet time
6. Postoperative management
  (i) Can be done as a day case surgery
  (ii) Encourage early activity and keep elevated
7. Complications
  Division of
  a. Superficial cutaneous branch of median nerve
  b. Recurrent motor branch of median nerve to thenar eminence

EXCISION OF DUPUYTREN'S CONTRACTURE

1. Indications
Incapacitating Dupuytrens contracture
2. Preoperative management
Examine and mark the side
3. Pre-incision
  (i) General anaesthetic
  (ii) Position
    Supine with arm extended on a side table
  (iii) Exsanguinate the arm with and inflate an arm tourniquet to a pressure of 250 mmHg, *note the time*
  (iv) Skin preparation of all of hand and forearm
4. Incision
  (i) Mark out a zig-zag incision commencing proximal to the contracture on the palm and extending distal to the contracture on the finger
  (ii) Incise the skin and dissect off the contracture beneath the incision until normal palmar fascia is reached

5. Procedure
    (i) Commencing proximally, dissect the abnormal palmar
        fascia off the deeper structures and continue distally
        into the finger
    (ii) Divide any adhesions to the fibrous flexor sheath
    (iii) *Beware damage to the palmar digital neurovascular
         bundles*
6. Closure
    (i) Only drain if dissection is extensive
    (ii) Close the skin loosely
    (iii) Large, firm padded bandage
7. Postoperative management
    Keep elevated for several days and encourage early activity
8. Complications
    Operative
    a. Severe finger flexion contracture, either excise the volar
       capsule or if severely incapacitating obtain conset for
       amputation
    b. Damage to neurovascular bundle

TREATMENT OF HAND INFECTIONS

1. Superficial
    (i) (95%)
        a. Paronychia
        b. Subcutaneous abscess
        c. Pulp space infection (Whitlow)
        d. Web space
        e. Middle volar infection (may spread and become deep)
    (ii) Treatment
        a. Direct incision to drain pus which should be sent for
           microbiological examination
        b. Appropriate antibiotics for a full therapeutic course
        c. Keep hand elevated
2. Deep
    (i) (5%)
    (ii) Clinically
        a. Swollen throbbing painful hand
        b. Systemically unwell
        c. Greatly diminished movement in hand
    (iii) Suppurating tenosynovitis
        a. Single sheath
        b. Ulnar bursa
        c. Radial bursa
        d. Full therapeutic course of flucloxacillin
        e. Drain synovial sheath both *proximally and distally* and
           irrigate the sheath with antibiotic solution

f. Elevate and encourage early mobilisation to reduce fibrous adhesions within the sheath
- (iv) Fascial space infection
    - a. Lateral (thenar) space
        Incise 1st web posteriorly
    - b. Medial (palmar) space
        Incise directly
    - c. Hypothenar space
        Incise directly
    - d. All incisions in skin creases
    - e. Divide tissues *longitudinally* thereby avoiding neurovascular bundles, tendons etc
    - f. Trim skin edges
    - g. Elevate and encourage early mobilisation
- (v) Complications
    - a. Infection
        Septicaemia
        Lymphangitis
        Spread via space of Parona to forearm
    - b. Suppurative arthritis
        Median nerve compression
        Stiff fingers
    - c. Persistent suppuration
        Foreign body
        Other sheath/space involved
        Osteomyelitis
        Sloughed tendon

LUMBAR LAMINECTOMY

1. Indications
    - (i) Immediate
        - a. Acute central disc protrusion
        - b. Acute lateral disc protrusion with lower motor neurone paralysis/sensory deficit
    - (ii) Urgent
        - a. Acute lateral disc protrusion
        - b. Extradural or intradural spinal tumour
        - c. Extradural abscess of the spine
    - (iii) After conservative management
        - a. Chronic disc protrusion
        - b. Lumbar spinal stenosis
2. Preoperative management
    - (i) Full, documented neurological examination
    - (ii) Investigations
        - a. Plain X-rays — AP and lateral of all of the spine
        - b. Myelography

     (iii) IVI
     (iv) Broad spectrum antibiotics prophylaxis
3. Pre-incision
     (i) General anaesthesia with endotracheal intubation
     (ii) Position
        Prone, with chest and pelvis supported and lumbar
        spine flexed
     (iii) Skin preparation of all of back, towelled up to expose
        and midline over the lumbar spine
4. Incision
Longitudinal 12 cm midline centred on the affected disc
space
5. Procedure
     (i) Deepen the incision to the spinous processes and clean
        the erector spinae muscles off the spinous processes
        and laminae on the side of the lesion with cutting
        diathermy
     (ii) Insert a self retaining retractor
     (iii) Identify the sacrum which moves with the pelvis and
        then the lamina overlying the compressed root by
        counting up from L5/S1 above the sacrum
     (iv) Excise the lower half of the lamina above with bone
        nibblers
     (v) Pick up and excise the ligamentum flavum, bounded by
        the bony margins
     (vi) Identify and retract the dura medially to expose the
        prolapsed disc
     (vii) Extract the prolapsed disc and currette the disc space
     (viii) Ensure the nerve root now lies free in its foramen
6. Closure
     (i) No drains
     (ii) Close — Lumbar fascia
               Skin
7. Postoperative management
Encourage early mobilisation with adequate analgesia
8. Investigations
     (i) If for abscess
        Pus for microscopy, culture and sensitivity
     (ii) If for tumour
        Histological examination
9. Complications
     (i) Early
        a. Ileus
        b. Acute retention
     (ii) Late
        Recurrent disc if curettage is inadequate

APPROACH TO THE HIP JOINT

1. Preoperation
   (i) Examine and mark side
   (ii) Investigations
       a. X-ray of hip — AP
                          Lateral
   (iii) Broad spectrum antibiotic prophylaxis
2. Pre-incision
   General anaesthesia with endotracheal intubation

A. Posterior approach
   (i) Position
       Lateral with pillow between legs
   (ii) Skin preparation loin to knee with U drape in groin and leg towelled separately
1. Incision
   20 cm long centred on greater trochanter curved superiorly towards posterior superior iliac spine
2. Procedure
   (i) Deepen incision including fascia/ilio tibial tract
   (ii) Divide insertion of gluteus maximus to posterior aspect of greater trochanter separating anterior border to gluteus maximus from gluteus medius
   (iii) Divide insertions of
       a. Obturator internus with gemelli
       b. Quadratus femoris
          and reflect posteriorly — thereby protecting the sciatic nerve lying posteriorly
   (iv) *Beware sciatic nerve posteriorly*
   (v) Perform capsulotomy
   (vi) Incise the exposed capsule and dislocate hip with internal rotation and flexion with adduction

B. Anterior approach
   (i) Position
       Supine
   (ii) Skin preparation of loin to knee, U drape to perineum and towel up with leg free
1. Incision
   Anterior superior iliac spine to greater trochanter and continue laterally 10 cm along thigh
2. Procedure
   (i) Deepen incision to fascia lata/ilio tibial tract
   (ii) Deepen between sartorius and tensor fascia lata, dividing origin of sartorius
   (iii) *Beware lateral circumflex iliac vessels*
   (iv) Divide origin of rectus femoris near anterior superior iliac spine to display capsule

  (v) Perform capsulotomy
  (vi) Dislocate hip with external rotation
3. Closure
    (i) Drain
        a. To joint
        b. To wound
    (ii) Close in layers

TOTAL HIP REPLACEMENT

1. Indications
    (i) Osteoarthritis
    (ii) Rheumatoid arthritis
2. Preoperative management
    (i) Exclude sites of chronic sepsis
    (ii) Examine and mark the side
    (iii) Broad spectrum antibiotic prophylaxis intravenously with
          induction achieves best bone levels
    (iv) IVI
    (v) Catheterise if appropriate
3. Pre-incision
   As for approach to the hip (see page 173), either approach
   is acceptable
4. Procedure
    (i) Perform capsulotomy and dislocate the joint
    (ii) Excise the joint capsule
    (iii) Divide the femoral neck in a line obliquely 1–2 cm
          above the greater trochanter. Cut the ligamentum teres
          to remove the head
    (iv) Ream the acetabulum down to bone until it is large
         enough to accept the acetabular prosthesis
    (v) Drill two or three keyholes in the acetabulum (one into
        each of the ilium, ischium and pubis)
    (vi) Prepare the methyl meth-acrylate bone cement and fix
         the acetabular component
    (vii) Prepare further bone cement and fix the femoral
          component
    (viii) Reduce the hip
5. Closure
   As for approach to the hip (see pages 173–174)
6. Postoperative management
    (i) Investigation
        Check X-rays of reduction
    (ii) Mobilise after 2 days
7. Complications
    (i) Operative
        a. Fracture of femoral shaft

b. Penetration of acetabulum into pelvis
c. Wrong acetabular geometry allowing post-reduction dislocation
d. Hypotension with implantation of cement
(ii) Postoperative
a. Infection — May result in loosening
Salvage with Girdlestones operation
b. Loosening — Infection
Reduce with high pressure cement injections
c. Calcification in soft tissues around prosthesis

MEDIAL MENISCECTOMY

1. Preoperative preparation
   (i) Examine and mark the side
   (ii) Commence quadriceps exercises
   (iii) Negro needs Sickle test for tourniquet
   (iv) X-rays/arthrograms of knee
   (v) Arthroscopy
2. Pre-incision
   (i) General anaesthetic with endotracheal intubation
   Exsanguinate leg and apply a tourniquet to affected thigh at 500 mmHg pressure and *note time*
   (ii) Position
   Supine with legs unsupported below the flexed knees
   (iii) Skin preparation of upper thigh to ankle with lower leg towelled separately and knee draped in op-site or sterile tubular bandage
   (iv) Surgeon
   Seated facing affected knee with the foot in his lap
3. Incision
   Vertical, medial to patella and its tendon from above knee to level with tibial tubercle
4. Procedure
   (i) Incise capsule in the line of the incision and retract medially
   (ii) Assess
      a. Medial meniscus
      b. Joint — Loose bodies
      c. Osteochondritis
      d. Arthritic changes
   (iii) Divide anterior horn, grasping meniscus with Kocher's forceps
   (iv) Divide capsular attachment with a Smillie knife
   (v) Detach posterior horn by sharp dissection

5. Closure
   (i) Haemostasis
       Release some of tourniquet pressure to check
   (ii) Close in layers
   (iii) Dress: either
        a. POP back slab
        b. Modified Robert Jones bandage
6. Postoperative care
   (i) Commence straight leg raising/quadriceps exercises next
       day
   (ii) If possible then commence walking, non weight bearing,
        at 2–3 days
7. Complications
   (i) Infection
   (ii) Haemarthrosis

KELLER'S OPERATION FOR HALLUX VALGUS

1. Indications
   Disabling hallux valgus with severe pain
2. Preoperative management
   (i) Examine and mark the side
   (ii) Investigations
        a. X-rays of foot
        b. Sickle status in Negroes prior to tourniquet
3. Pre-incision
   (i) General anaesthetic
   (ii) Position
        Supine
   (iii) Exsanguinate the leg with and inflate a thigh tourniquet
         to 500 mmHg, *note the time*
   (iv) Skin preparation of foot and lower leg
4. Incision
   5 cm longitudinally directly over bunion
5. Procedure
   (i) Deepen the incision down to bone
   (ii) Dissect out the bursa over the medial metatarsal head,
        opening the joint capsule medially
   (iii) Grasp the proximal phallanx and cut off the proximal
         1 cm with a bone cutter
   (iv) With a narrow osteotome, excise the medial exostosis of
        the metatarsal head
6. Closure
   (i) Close the joint capsule with absorbable sutures
   (ii) Close the skin and apply a firm support dressing to the
        hallux and rest of foot
   (iii) Release the tourniquet, documenting the tourniquet time
         and checking the return of circulation to the toes

7. Postoperative management
   (i) Encourage early mobilisation, non weight bearing
   (ii) Ordinary shoes can be worn after about 3 months
8. Complications
   (i) Hallux dorsiflexion deformity
       Needs lengthening plastic procedure of extensor hallucis longus
   (ii) Persistent valgus deformity
       Fix the truncated proximal phallanx to the metatarsal head with a longitudinal Kirschner wire to encourage fibrous ankylosis in that position

ZADEK'S OPERATION

1. Indications
   Chronic ingrowing great toe nail
2. Contraindications
   (i) Sepsis
   (ii) Peripheral vascular disease
3. Preoperative management
   (i) Examine and mark the side
   (ii) Exclude diabetes as a contributory factor in recurrent infection
4. Pre-incision
   (i) Either general or local ring block (*Avoid adrenaline*) anaesthesia
   (ii) Position
       Supine
   (iii) Skin preparation of all of foot, apply a rubber tourniquet to the proximal hallux
5. Procedure
   (i) Remove the toe nail
   (ii) Make two oblique incisions into the skin at each corner of the nail bed for 0.5–1 cm
   (iii) Retract the skin off the germinal matrix of the nail root for the whole of its width
   (iv) Excise the nail matrix underlying the skin for its whole width down to periostium
   (v) *Beware leaving pockets of nail matrix in each corner*
6. Closure
   (i) Suture the two skin incisions
   (ii) Dress the wound with a non-adherent dressing
   (iii) Release the tourniquet and check re-establishment of the circulation
7. Postoperative management
   This can be done as day case surgery
8. Complications
   Recurrent ingrowth of spikes of nail left from residual germinal matrix in the corners

SITES OF MAJOR JOINT ASPIRATION

1. Wrist
   Posteriorly, between extensor pollicis longus and extensor indicis
2. Elbow
   (i) Postero laterally
       Above radial head
   (ii) Posteriorly
       In midline
3. Shoulder
   Anteriorly by medial border of deltoid (avoid cephalic vein)
4. Hip
   (i) Anteriorly
       2.5 cm below and lateral to mid inguinalpoint (beware femoral artery and nerve)
   (ii) Laterally
       Just above the tip of the greater trochanter, then pass upwards and medially over the femoral neck
5. Knee
   Either medial or lateral to patellar tendon
6. Ankle
   Anterior to lateral malleolus
7. Investigations
   (i) If for abscess
       Pus for microscopy, culture and sensitivity
   (ii) If for gout
       Microscopy for crystals

Trauma surgery

LAPAROTOMY FOR ABDOMINAL TRAUMA

1. Resuscitate
   (i) Airway
   (ii) Breathing
   (iii) Circulation — Peripheral IVIs
       a. At least two cannulae
       b. Cross match at least 6 units of blood urgently
2. Assess
   (i) Catheterise
       Haematuria: proceed to IVP with continuous Conray
       infusion (see principles of urological trauma
       management, page 186)
   (ii) Rectal examination
   (iii) Plain abdominal X-rays
       a. Foreign bodies
       b. Free gas
   (iv) Beware effects of cavitation shock waves transmitted by
       the great vessels following high velocity missile injuries
       to limbs
   (v) Peritoneal lavage is approx. 90% accurate in detecting
       significant intraperitoneal haemorrhage (false positive
       rate 2–3%)
   (vi) Careful repeated observations
3. Indications for laparotomy
   (i) All penetrating wounds (no matter how superficial they
       appear in the casualty department)
   (ii) Blunt abdominal trauma
       a. Hypovolaemic shock
       b. Free gas on plain abdominal X-rays
       c. Clothing imprintation on the skin
       d. Peritonism
       e. Blood stained peritoneal lavage

(iii) *Beware concomittant major injury*
  a. *Pelvic fracture*
  b. *Chest (see management of major chest trauma, page 182) — Flail segment*
      — Adult respiratory distress syndrome
        Intrapleural tension
  c. *Head*
4. Pre-procedure
  (i) In profound hypovolaemia, do not delay surgery in an attempt to restore the blood pressure
  (ii) Broad spectrum and metronidazole antibiotic cover
  (iii) Antitetanus measures
5. Pre-incision
  (i) General anaesthesia and endotracheal intubation, induced once the patient is on the operating table
    a. Central venous pressure monitor ⎫ Can wait until surgery
    b. Arterial line ⎭ is underway
  (ii) Position
    a. Supine
    b. Upper abdominal trauma — Consider thoraco-abdominal approach
  (iii) Skin preparation of all of abdomen from above the nipples to mid thigh
6. Incision
  Excise and close penetrating wound, then proceed to laparotomy
7. Procedure
  (i) Needs full laparotomy
  (ii) Profuse bleeding
    a. Evacuate clots
    b. Systematically pack off all four quadrants with large abdominal swabs and then remove to localise the source of the bleeding
  (iii) Kocherise the duodenum
    a. Posterior duodenum
    b. Posterior head of pancreas
    c. IVC
    d. Right renal area
  (iv) Open both lateral colic peritoneal reflections to examine the posterior ascending and descending colon
  (v) Examine the pelvis
    a. Urological trauma (see page 186)

b. Rectal injury — Drain pelvis
Proximal colostomy
Drain presacral area by excising
coccyx

Injury to specific organs
1. Small bowel and mesentery
   (i) Perforation
      a. Small — Repair
      b. Large — Resect
   (ii) Mesenteric tear: Transverse — Resect
   As vessels often involved: Longitudinal — Repair
2. Large bowel
   (i) *Avoid primary resection with anastomosis*
   (ii) Caecum
      a. Right hemicolectomy with ileostomy and mucous
      fistula
      b. Transverse/descending colon — Excise with proximal
      colostomy and mucous fistula
3. Liver
   (i) Profuse bleeding
   Pringle's manoeuvre (pinch hepatic artery and portal vein
   in right free border of lesser omentum)
   (ii) See hepatic resection (page 111)
4. Spleen
   (i) Small tear — Consider repair and preservation
   (ii) Large tear — Splenectomy (see page 105)
5. Retroperitoneum
   (i) Duodenum
      a. Kocherise and examine fully
      b. Repair and drain perforation
   (ii) Pancreas
      a. Head — Small — Drain
             Large — Consider resection
      b. Tail — Small — Drain
             Large — Resect with spleen
   (iii) Haematoma
      a. Small — Leave
      b. Large — Evacuate and drain
   (iv) Kidney (see urological trauma, page 186)
6. Problems
   (i) Severe uncontrollable pelvic bleeding — consider
   angiography and embolisation of pelvic vessels
   (ii) Severe liver injury
      a. May need right thoracotomy to control caval bleeding
      b. Transfer to regional hepatobiliary unit

7. Multiple injuries
   (i) 10% have abdominal injuries — 25% mortality
     a. Of these 10% — 30% have thoracic   — 40% mortality
                    injuries
                    30% have pelvic   30% mortality
                    injuries
                    30% have leg   30% mortality
                    injuries
                    20% have head   50% mortality
                    injuries
     b. Major abdominal, chest and head injury — 80% mortality
   (ii) Consider tracheostomy (see page 54)
8. Postoperative management
   (i) Once stable, transfer to regional trauma/specialist unit if necessary
   (ii) Nurse on an intensive care unit
   (iii) Monitor
     a. Pulse
     b. Blood pressure
     c. CVP
     d. Urine output
     e. Packed cell volume/haemoglobin and transfuse accordingly
9. Complications
   (i) Acute renal failure
   (ii) Adult respiratory distress syndrome
   (iii) Infection
     a. Peritonitis
     b. Wound
     c. Abscess
     d. Septicaemia
     e. Respiratory tract
     f. *Clostridia*
   (iv) Disseminated intravascular coagulation
   (v) Upper gastrointestinal bleeding

MANAGEMENT OF MAJOR CHEST TRAUMA

1. Resuscitate
   (i) Airway
   (ii) Breathing
   (iii) Circulation
     a. At least two IVIs
     b. Cross match 10 units of blood
   (iv) Drain to relieve tension
     a. Pleura
     b. Pericardium
   (v) Excise and close wounds

2. Management
   (i) 90% of blunt chest trauma can be managed
       conservatively
   (ii) 80% of penetrating chest wounds can be managed by
        excision and primary wound closure with underwater
        seal drainage if penetrating beyond parietal pleura
3. Problems
   (i) Penetrating wounds frequently do not occur in isolation
   (ii) Chest and neck
       a. Brachial plexus
       b. Carotid sheath structures
       c. Thoracic duct on left
       d. Trachea/oesophagus
   (iii) Chest and abdomen
        needs thoracoabdominal exposure (see laparotomy for
        abdominal trauma, page 179)
   (iv) Blunt injuries
       a. Concomittent spinal and pelvic injury
       b. Head injury (see craniotomy for extradural
          haematoma, page 192)
       c. Abdominal injury (see laparotomy for abdominal
          trauma, page 179)
4. Specific intrathoracic problems
   (i) Great vessels, especially with crushing chest injury (see
       vascular trauma management, page 184)
   (ii) Chest wall: flail/stove in injury, manage with positive
        pressure ventilation and wiring of ribs
   (ii) Pleura
       a. Pneumothorax — Simple
                           Tension
       b. Haemothorax — Usually from intercostal vessels
   (iii) Pericardial tamponade
   (iv) Direct myocardial damage — Needs 12-lead ECG
   (v) Trachea/main bronchus fracture — Repair
5. Exploration
   (i) Use posterolateral thoracotomy (see page 68)
   (ii) Never use positive pressure ventilation when there is a
        suspicion of pneumothorax until pleural drains are in
        place
   (iii) Indications for thoracotomy
       a. Excessive uncontrollable bleeding
       b. Excessive air leak from broncho-pleural fistula
       c. Penetrating wound to mediastinum/pericardium
       d. Tamponade
       e. Thoracoabdominal injury
       f. Chest wall defect
   (iv) Relative indications for thoracotomy
        sucking chest wall wound

     (v) Antibiotic cover
        a. Broad spectrum and flucloxacillin
        b. Tetanus cover
    (vi) Consider transfer to regional cardiothoracic centre once
        stable

VASCULAR TRAUMA MANAGEMENT

1. Assessment
   (i) *Always suspect*
       a. All limb injuries especially fractures of long bones
       b. Enlarging/pulsating haematoma
       c. Distal vascular insufficiency (diminished pulse or
          Doppler pressure)
   (ii) Manage life threatening problems before limb
        threatening problems
   (iii) Venous injury is as important as arterial injury
   (iv) Clinical examination of arteries
        a. Pulses
        b. Pressure — Auscultation
                           Doppler
        c. Evidence of ischaemic anaesthesia
   (v) Presence of Doppler arterial pulse does *not* exclude
       arterial disruption
   (vi) X-rays
        a. Plain in two planes at 90° to each other — Fracture
                                             Foreign
                                             body
        b. Arteriogram when in doubt about presence of, or site
           of, arterial injury
   (vii) *Never ascribe arterial disruption to spasm*
2. Principles of management
   (i) Control haemorrhage
       Direct pressure
   (ii) Prevent infection
        a. Antisepsis, debridement, antitetanus
        b. Broad spectrum antibiotic with flucloxacillin
   (iii) Stabilise fracture
         Consider indwelling shunt in artery if delay likely
   (iv) Restore circulation
        a. General anaesthetic
        b. Good exposure of injury
        c. Good control of arteries and veins both proximally
           and distally
        d. Evacuate haematoma
   (v) Repair
       Options
       a. End-to-end anastomosis of divided vessels; suture of
          incised injury

    b. Vein patch over defect
    c. Extensive defect — Insert reverse vein graft (vein
       from *uninjured* limb)
 (vi) Local anticoagulation with heparin in saline (5000 units
      in 500 ml normal saline)
(vii) *Reassess veins after restoring arterial supply*
    a. Debride wound
    b. Cover arterial repair
    c. Do not close contaminated wounds
3. Indications for fasciotomy
  (i) Extensive soft tissue damage
 (ii) Swelling
(iii) > 6 hours delay after injury/embolism
 (iv) Combined arterio-venous injury
  (v) Any popliteal vessel trauma

  (i) Decompress all compartments (in the leg this can be
      achieved by fibula excision)
 (ii) *Volkmanns type of ischaemia will occur with a tissue
      hydrostatic pressure of > 50 mmHg, and therefore can
      arise in the presence of palpable peripheral pulses*
(iii) Postoperatively
      Needs regular review of ischaemic limb, re-explore if
      any evidence of diminishing circulation

Specific arterial problems
1. Thoracic aorta
    (i) Decelleration injuries (car driver)
   (ii) Usually between left subclavian artery and ligamentum
        arteriosum
  (iii) 20% will survive to reach hospital and may have good
        equal femoral pulses
   (iv) Investigations
      a. Diagnosis *on suspicion* from the history
      b. CXR — Widening aorta
              Depressed left main bronchus
              NG tube displaced to right
      c. Arch aortogram
    (v) Preoperative neurological examination of legs
   (vi) Proceed to surgery in a cardiac unit if possible,
        therefore cardio-pulmonary bypass feasible
  (vii) Simple bypass is possible with a silastic catheter
        between the apex of the left ventricle and
        descending aorta
 (viii) *Beware associated injuries*
      a. Myocardial contusion
      b. Adult respiratory distress syndrome
      c. Multiple injuries
      d. Paraplegia due to spinal cord ischaemia

2. Femoral artery — Often occurs in association with venous injury
   (i) Common femoral
       Rare
       a. Penetrating — Butchers knife
       b. orthopaedic procedure
   (ii) Superficial femoral
       a.   Common — Fractured femur
       b.   Treatment — Ligation — 50% amputation rate
                        Repair — 10% amputation rate
3. Popliteal artery — 60% have associated popliteal vein injury
   (i) Associated with
       a. Direct trauma
       b. Knee dislocation
       c. Menisectomy
   (ii) Repair artery and reconstruct veins
        < 20% amputation
   (iii) Ligate artery
        80% amputation rate
   (iv) Always requires full length, four compartment fasciotomy
4. Brachial artery — *Common iatrogenic injury*
   (Following cardiac catheterisation)
   (i) Associated nerve injury
       a. Ischaemic
       b. Direct trauma to median and ulnar nerve
   (ii) *Always reconstruct*

PRINCIPLES OF UROLOGICAL TRAUMA MANAGEMENT

A.   Renal trauma
 1. Establish diagnosis
    (i) History
        a. Blunt trauma
        b. Penetrating injury
    (ii) Examination
        a. Bruising/laceration
        b. Haematoma
        c. *Haematuria*
    (iii) Associated injury
        a. fractured ribs
        b. Spleen/liver (see splenectomy, page 105 and principles of hepatic resection, page 111) and lung (see management of major chest trauma, page 182)
        c. Spine

(iv) Abdominal X-ray
    a. Loss or renal/psoas shadow
    b. Fractured lower ribs
    c. Protective scoliosis
    d. Soft tissue mass (haematoma)
2. Antibiotics
  Broad spectrum
3. IVU by continuous Conray infusion
5. Management

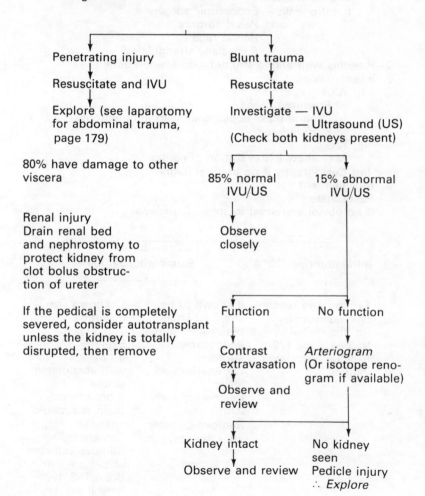

Penetrating injury

Resuscitate and IVU

Explore (see laparotomy
for abdominal trauma,
page 179)

80% have damage to other
viscera

Renal injury
Drain renal bed
and nephrostomy to
protect kidney from
clot bolus obstruc-
tion of ureter

If the pedical is completely
severed, consider autotransplant
unless the kidney is totally
disrupted, then remove

Blunt trauma

Resuscitate

Investigate — IVU
           — Ultrasound (US)
(Check both kidneys present)

85% normal   15% abnormal
IVU/US   IVU/US

Observe
closely

Function   No function

Contrast   *Arteriogram*
extravasation (Or isotope reno-
              gram if available)

Observe and
review

Kidney intact   No kidney
                seen
Observe and review Pedicle injury
                ∴ *Explore*

B.   Bladder trauma
1. Establish diagnosis
    (i) *Blunt trauma*
        a. Direct blow to full bladder usually causes
            intraperitoneal rupture
        b. Fractured pelvis (beware associated urethural injury)
            may cause extraperitoneal rupture
    (ii) Penetrating injury
        a. Stab wound
        b. Iatrogenic — Endoscopic surgery
                         Pelvic surgery
                         Hernia repair
                         (Especially strangulated)
2. Presents with anuria/scanty blood stained urine
3. Investigations
    (i) AXR
        a. Fractured pelvis
        b. Ground glass appearance with intraperitoneal
            perforation
    (ii) IVU
        May show extravasation of contrast
    (iii) Cystography if no urethral injury
4. Management
    Resuscitate
    If no obvious urethral injury — Catheterise

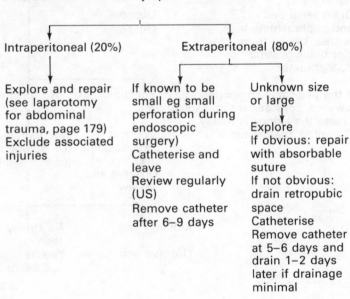

Intraperitoneal (20%)   Extraperitoneal (80%)

Explore and repair   If known to be   Unknown size
(see laparotomy   small eg small   or large
for abdominal   perforation during
trauma, page 179)   endoscopic   Explore
Exclude associated   surgery)   If obvious: repair
injuries   Catheterise and   with absorbable
                        leave   suture
                        Review regularly   If not obvious:
                        (US)   drain retropubic
                        Remove catheter   space
                        after 6–9 days   Catheterise
                                              Remove catheter
                                              at 5–6 days and
                                              drain 1–2 days
                                              later if drainage
                                              minimal

C. Male urethral injuries

1. Establish diagnosis
   - (i) History of either fall astride injury (bulbar urethra) or pelvic injury (membranous urethra) with inability to pass urine (beware neurogenic acute retention with concomittant spinal injury)
   - (ii) Inability to pass urine after traumatic endoscopic surgery
   - (iii) Blood at external meatus ± perineal bruising
   - (iv) Beware associated bladder injury
2. Investigations
   - (i) Plain pelvic X-rays
   - (ii) IVU
   - (iii) *Avoid urethrogram*
     - a. may convert an incomplete rupture into a complete rupture
   - (iv) An experienced urologist may try one attempt to pass a fine, soft urethral catheter into the bladder
3. Urinary extravasation
   - (i) Prostatic urethral injury
     - a. Deep to muscles of anterior abdominal wall and triangular ligament
     - b. Within fascia of Denonvilliers
   - (ii) Bulbar urethral injury
     - a. Deep to Scarpa's fascia
     - b. Within Colles fascia
4. Management — See page 190

PRINCIPLES OF MANAGEMENT OF LIMB WOUNDS

1. Assess
   - (i) All pulses
   - (ii) Nerves
     - a. Motor
     - b. Sensory
   - (iii) *Beware missile injuries with only small entry wounds causing cavitation effects and destroying collateral circulation* (see laparotomy for abdominal trauma, page 179)
   - (iv) Investigations
     - a. Plain X-rays in at least two planes including joint above and joint below
     - b. Arteriography if vascular injury suspected (see vascular trauma management, page 184)
   - (v) Full antimicrobial prophylaxis
     - a. Antitetanus measures
     - b. Broad spectrum antibiotics and flucloxacillin with penicillin for clostridia

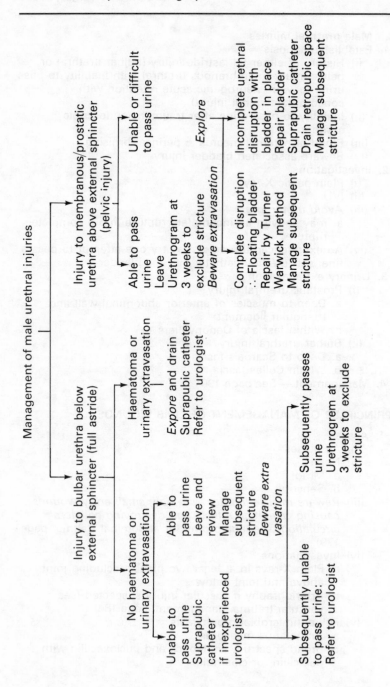

Management of male urethral injuries

Injury to membranous/prostatic urethra above external sphincter (pelvic injury)

Able to pass urine
Leave
Urethrogram at 3 weeks to exclude stricture
Beware extravasation

Unable or difficult to pass urine
Explore

Complete disruption
∴ Floating bladder
Repair by Turner Warwick method
Manage subsequent stricture

Incomplete urethral disruption with bladder in place
Repair bladder
Suprapubic catheter
Drain retropubic space
Manage subsequent stricture

Injury to bulbar urethra below external sphincter (fall astride)

Haematoma or urinary extravasation
Explore and drain
Suprapubic catheter
Refer to urologist

No haematoma or urinary extravasation

Able to pass urine
Leave and review
Manage subsequent stricture
Beware extravasation

Unable to pass urine
Suprapubic catheter if inexperienced urologist

Subsequently passes urine
Urethrogram at 3 weeks to exclude stricture

Subsequently unable to pass urine:
Refer to urologist

c. Aseptic techniques
d. Antiseptics with full debridement (*Avoid alcohol* — May irreparably damage nerves and tendons)

2. Procedure
   Needs
   a. Good regional or general anaesthesia
   b. good exposure — Using longitudinal incisions *and preserving skin*
   c. Good light

3. Vascular injuries (see vascular trauma management, page 184)
   (i) Always reconstruct both arteries and veins
   (ii) *Beware high velocity missile injury destroying collateral circulation*
   (iii) Always needs full length fasciotomies

4. Nerves (see principles of management of nerve and tendon injury, page 199)
   (i) Simple laceration — Primary repair if possible
   (ii) Otherwise label with nonabsorbable suture and close; attempt delayed primary repair at 6 weeks

5. Muscle
   (i) If viability doubtful — *Excise*
   (ii) Prevent
       a. Infection (especially gas gangrene)
       b. Contractures (ischaemia, immobility)

6. Tendons (see principles of management of nerve and tendon injury, page 199)
   (i) Single
       Consider repair
   (ii) Multiple
        Label with nonabsorbable sutures for delayed repair after skin cover completed

7. Bone
   (i) Preserve all fragments, curreting and scraping out any debris
   (ii) Irrigate with antiseptic solution
   (iii) *Beware internal fixation with compound fractures*

8. Joints
   (i) Exposure needs tourniquet control
   (ii) Remove all debris with debridement
   (iii) Irrigate
   (iv) Always close synovium (substitute muscle or skin if synovium lost)

9. At end
   (i) Liberally apply antiseptic soaked dressings
   (ii) Never close if any risk of contamination or with gunshot wounds
   (iii) *Elevate*

10. Traumatic amputation
    (i) Guillotine
        Consider reimplantation
    (ii) Avulsion/ragged transection
        a. Needs total debridement
        b. Leave open — Allows drainage
                        Protect skin edges
        c. Delayed primary closure
11. Hand/foot
    (i) Fully decompress and debride wound
    (ii) Leave open and elevate until all swelling reduced
    (iii) Then close/skin graft as soon as possible
12. If wound left open
    (i) Examine under anaesthetic on the fifth day, if clean,
        consider closure/skin grafts
    (ii) Never close under tension

CRANIOTOMY FOR EXTRADURAL HAEMATOMA

1. Preoperative management
    (i) Informed consent from relative
    (ii) Investigations
        a. Skull X-rays
        b. CT scan
        c. (Ultrasound)
    (iii) Preparation
        Shave head completely
    (iv) Antibiotics
        Benzyl penicillin/sulphonamides
    (v) IVI (beware fluid overload)
    (vi) Catheterise
    (vii) NG tube (both for aspiration and postoperative feeding)
    (viii) Endotracheal tube, preoperatively $\uparrow$ PaO_2 and $\downarrow$ PaCO_2
        by hyperventilation to reduce intracranial pressure
2. Pre-incision
    (i) General anaesthesia with endotracheal intubation
    (ii) *Avoid inhalation anaesthetic gases*
        especially HALOTHANE since they increase intracranial
        pressure
    (iii) Position
        Supine
3. Incision
    (i) Preauricular: from zygoma to above temple, deepen
        through all layers to pericranium
    (ii) Separate fibres of temporalis
    (iii) *Avoid facial nerve* — Especially temporal branch

4. Procedure
   (i) Insert self restraining retractor and visualise fracture in superficial temporal bone
   (ii) Commence burr anterior to fracture line with 16 mm Hudson brace to superficial table and with burr to inner table
   (iii) Extradural haematoma should now be visible
   (iv) Extend burr hole with bone nibblers to beyond edge of haematoma
   (v) Remove haematoma from the edge first with sucker (clearing clot from junction of bone and dura)
   (vi) The intracranial pressure should decrease and the clot commence to pulsate as the arterial circulation improves
   (vii) As the clot is removed, the intracranial pressure continues to decrease and the bleeding correspondingly increases
   (viii) Remove centre of clot over bleeding point on middle meningeal artery and ligate with a non-absorbable suture (beware catching the middle cerebral artery lying immediately below the dura with this suture!)
5. Complications
   (i) Burr reveals no haematoma but bulging dura — Do not open further since results in cerebral herniation
   (ii) Either do exploratory burrs around cranium or better
   (iii) Refer for CT scan
6. Closure
   (i) Suture dura to temporalis muscle all around edge of craniectomy
   (ii) Haemostasis
   (iii) Close scalp in layers
   (iv) *If tracheostomy necessary, best to perform immediately* (see page 54)
7. Postoperative management
   (i) Quarter-hourly neurological observation
   (ii) Ventilate to maintain
       a. High PaO_2
       b. Low $PaCO_2$
   (iii) Tracheostomy/endotracheal tube care
   (iv) Physiotherapy (chest and passive limb movement), intensive nursing care
   (v) Continue antibiotics for one week
   (vi) Investigation
       If dura opened: daily lumbar puncture for microbiological examination

MANAGEMENT OF FRACTURE NECK OF FEMUR

1. Preoperative management
   (i) Examine and mark the side
   (ii) Investigations
       Plain X-rays of hip — AP
                            Lateral
   (iii) Establish the site of fracture
       a. Subcapital
       b. Neck
       c. Trochanteric
   (iv) Catheterise
   (v) IVI
   (vi) Broad spectrum antibiotic prophylaxis intravenously at
       induction achieves highest bone levels
2. Pre-incision
   either general anaesthesia with endotracheal intubation or
   spinal anaesthesia

A. **Trochanteric and undisplaced subcapital (Garden I and II)
   fracture of the femur**
   (i) Position
       a. Supine on an orthopaedic operating table abducting
          the good leg and reducing the fracture by traction,
          10° abduction and internal rotation to the affected leg
       b. set up X-ray image intensifier to be able to view the
          hip in both AP and lateral views
   (ii) Skin preparation from knee to upper abdomen
   (iii) Drape up to allow exposure to lateral upper thigh with
        access for image intensifier (Or use Fitzgerald polythene
        'sail')
1. Incision
   20 cm commencing posterior to greater trochanter and
   extending longitudinally down the thigh
2. Procedure
   (i) Divide fascia lata in the line of the incision
   (ii) Divide upper origin of vastus lateralis and separate
       from upper lateral femur
   (iii) Select a site on the lower posterior margin of the
        greater trochanter and cut a small hole in the cortex
   (iv) Pass two or more guide wires up through the fracture
        line along the posterior inferior part of the femoral neck
        to lie in the femoral head
   (v) *Beware guide wire penetration of the pelvis*
   (vi) Check the position of the guide wires with the image
        intensifier and select the best positioned. Measure the
        length of guide wire in bone and choose a nail 1 cm
        shorter

    (vii) Ream the cortex around the insertion of the guide wire
  (viii) Hammer in the selected nail (e.g. McLaughlin or
       McKee) along the guide wire
    (ix) Recheck the position of the nail radiologically
    (x) Clear the periostium off the lateral femoral shaft for
       15 cm
    (xi) Holding the plate to the femoral shaft, apply the plate
       to the butt of the nail. Secure the plate to the nail with
       the appropriate nut
    (xii) Secure the plate to the femoral shaft with at least 5
       screws through both cortices

3. Closure
    (i) Suction drain
    (ii) Close in layers

B. **Displaced subcapital (Garden III and IV) fractured neck of
femur**
    Needs hemiarthroplasty

1. Procedure
    (i) Needs full exposure of the hip joint (see page 173)
    (ii) Remove head of femur and measure to select suitable
       size of prosthesis
    (iii) Excise redundant neck of femur at greater trochanter
       and ream medulla for prosthesis (use either uncemented
       Austin Moore prosthesis or Thompson's prosthesis
       with cement)
    (iv) Insert prosthesis dry and perform trial reduction; then if
       necessary cement prosthesis
    (v) Reduce hip
    (vi) *Test stability*
    (vii) close according to approach (shown on page 173)

2. Postoperative management
    Encourage early mobilisation

3. Complications
    (i) Operative
       a. Nail plate method — Penetration of pelvis with nail
                          Damage to profunda femoris
                          with screws to plate
       b. Hemiarthroplasty — Fracture of femoral shaft during
         insertion of prosthesis
    (ii) Postoperative
       a. DVT
       b. Bronchopneumonia
       c. Dislocation of hemiarthroplasty
       d. Loosening of prosthesis

K-NAIL FOR FRACTURED FEMUR

1. Preoperative
   (i) Resuscitate
      a. Transfuse to correct hypovolaemia and haemoglobin
      b. Stabilise femur with traction [skin or skeletal with 20 lb (10 kg)]
   (ii) Examine and mark side
   (iii) Measure length of good femur (to choose length of nail) shave thigh and buttock
   (iv) Broad spectrum and flucloxacillin antibiotic prophylaxis
   (v) IVI
2. Pre-incision
   (i) Either spinal or general anaesthesia with endotracheal intubation
   (ii) Position
       Lateral
   (iii) Surgeon
       Posterior to patient
   (iv) Skin preparation
      a. Mid-abdomen, groin, buttock to below knee
      b. Thigh and buttock exposed
   (v) U-drape to perineum
3. Incisions
   (i) Lateral approach to mid-femur 20–30 cm in length
   (ii) Over greater trochanter
4. Procedure
   Mid thigh
   (i) Deepen between vastus lateralis and intermuscular septum
   (ii) Ligate perforating vessels
   (iii) Assess
      a. Fracture
      b. Soft tissue
      c. Fragments
      d. Reduce, assess stability
   (iv) *Beware sciatic nerve posteriorly*
   (v) Excessive traction to leg
       Ream upper fragments and measure medullary diameter to select width of nail
   (vi) Trochanteric incision
      a. Pass nail over guide wire through greater trochanter into upper fragment as far as fracture
      b. Ream lower fragment to femoral condyles
      c. Reduce fracture
      d. Pass nail the full length of the femur into the lower fragment

5. Closure
    (i) Suction drainage to both wounds
    (ii) Close in layers
6. Postoperative care
    (i) Investigation
        X-ray of femur
        a. Reduction
        b. Position of nail
    (ii) Mobilise gently
        a. Practise straight leg raising, walking, non-weight
           bearing with crutches at 1–2 weeks
        b. Weight bearing 4–6 weeks
        c. ? Remove nail at 12–18 months
7. Complications
    (i) Infection
        a. Nail
        b. Wounds
    (ii) Fracture
        a. Delayed union
        b. Non-union
        c. Mal union
        d. Nail displacement
    (iii) *DVT/PE* (see principles of prevention of DVT, page 7)

MANAGEMENT OF FRACTURED SHAFT OF TIBIA

A. Open fracture
    (i) Avoid closure
        a. Debride wound and antisepsis
        b. External fixation
    (ii) Broad spectrum antibiotic cover
    (iii) Antitetanus measure
    (iv) Examine under anaesthetic 5 days later, then close or
        graft skin if not infected

B. Closed fracture — Methods
1. Reduce with manipulation under anaesthesia
    (i) Place in a split plaster of Paris cast from mid thigh to
        mid tarsus, well padded with orthopaedic gauze
    (ii) Prevent rotation of fracture components
    (iii) *Monitor*
        a. *Swelling and distal circulation*
        b. *Displacement*
        c. *Union/consolidation*
    (iv) *Complication*
        a. *Compartment syndrome* — Needs fasciotomy
        b. Delayed/non union
        c. mal union

2. Os-calcis traction
   (i) With 10 lb (4 kg) traction via a Denham pin placed through the os calcis
   (ii) Support the leg on a pillow for 2 weeks
   (iii) Monitor
       a. Soft tissues
       b. Skin
       c. Peripheral circulation
       d. After 2 weeks either —   Internally fixate or
                                     cast brace
   (iv) Complications
       Subtalar joint stiffness
3. External fixation of the fragments
   (i) Allows
       a. Adjustment/compression of components
       b. Skin grafting
   (ii) Stability results in better soft tissue healing
   (iii) Complication
       Infection
4. Internal fixation
   Indication
   (i) Other injuries preclude above alternatives (eg femoral fracture)
   (ii) Old age — needs rapid mobilisation
   (iii) Irreducible/unholdable fracture
   (iv) Failure of above methods
   (v) Social (time in hospital/financial)

C. **Internal fixation of fractured tibia**
   (i) Protect leg by placing in skin or skeletal traction
   (ii) Mark the side
   (iii) Investigation
       X-rays of tibia including knee and ankle joint in two planes at right angles
   (iv) Preparation
       shave the leg
   (v) Broad spectrum and flucloxaillin antibiotic prophylaxis
1. Pre-incision
   (i) General anaesthetic
   (ii) *Avoid* tourniquet
   (iii) Position
       Supine
   (iv) Skin preparation of mid-thigh to foot
   (v) Towel up with skin exposed, foot covered but mobile
2. Incision
   Longitudinal along skin
3. Procedure
   (i) Elevate periosteum and display fracture line

(ii) Clean bone ends with minimal disturbance of callus and remove interposing soft tissues

(iii) Attempt reduction and brace fragements together

(iv) Position a template specific to fracture, sufficient to take at least four screws through both cortices in both proximal and distal fragments

(v) Adjust plate to the shape of the tibia and apply to bone, tapping screw holes

(vi) Screw the plate to the fragments with an optional screw through the fracture line if it is oblique

4. Closure
   (i) Suction drainage to plate
   (ii) Close in layers
       a. Periosteum over plate
       b. Skin
   (iii) Split P.O.P. cylinder (allows early mobilisation)

5. Postoperative care
   Check position of fragments on X-ray in two planes

6. Complications
   (i) Early
       a. Skin damage (especially lower third fracture)
       b. Infection
       c. Compartment syndrome (anterior compartment)
       d. Haematoma
   (ii) Late
       a. Fracture — Delayed or non-union especially with damaged nutrient artery to lower third
       b. Joint stiffness, if mobilisation delayed

PRINCIPLES OF MANAGEMENT OF NERVE AND TENDON INJURY

All lacerations need accurate assessment

1. Accurate history
   Position of hand at the time of injury since if in flexion with a flexor surface injury the tendons will retract

2. Management of sepsis is essential (see principles of prevention of surgical sepsis, page 4)
   (i) Mechanical cleansing
   (ii) Debridement
   (iii) Antisepsis
   (iv) Antitetatanus measures
       a. Passive
       b. Active
   (v) Antibiotics
       a. Topical
       b. Systemic

3. Exploration needs
   (i) Avascular field (tourniquet)
   (ii) Good light
   (iii) Adequate anaesthesia
   (iv) On table X-ray facilities
   (v) Wide exposure, converting laceration to a Z-incision
   (vi) Preserve all viable skin and aim to get primary skin cover, either closing without tension or by skin graft
4. Nerve injury
   (i) Digital nerves
   primary repair with epineural suture
   (ii) Major nerves — Indication to explore
       a. Open injury
       b. Closed injury with failure of recovery at expected rate of 100 mm in 100 days (follow with Tinnell's test)
       c. (NB: 90% of closed nerve injuries are neurapaxia)
5. Problem with major nerve repair
   (i) Arguments against primary repair
       a. Inexperience of surgeon
       b. Available facilities for micro-surgery
       c. Epineurium is very thin for the first 2 weeks
       d. Higher incidence of anastomotic neuroma
       e. Nature of injury and size of defect
   (ii) Therefore aim for initial skin cover and delayed repair; at 6 weeks there is good epineural tissue to suture and nerve viability can be more accurately assessed
6. Nerve repair
   (i) All nerve repairs should be performed after the tourniquet is released as an intraneural haematoma may jeopardise the repair
   (ii) Examine fascicles using the operating microscope as their arrangements change every centimetre
   (iii) Use 5/0 Prolene for epineural suture
   (iv) Consider cable nerve graft for a large defect of less than 10 cm, using greater auricular nerve as a donor
   (v) Ulnar nerve length can be gained by anterior transposition at the elbow (see ulnar nerve transposition, page 167)
   (vi) Support in plaster of Paris cast for 2 weeks
7. Tendon repair
   (i) Mallet finger
       a. Resisted extension injury either tearing the tendon or avulsing the base of the distal phalanx at the insertion of the extensor tendon
       b. 50% will recover after 4 weeks in a hyperextension splint

   (ii) Boutonniere
      a. Rupture of central slip of extensor tendon with
         subluxation of the interphalangeal joint
      b. Closed injury — Early reduction with hyperextension
         splint
      c. Open injury — Attempt repair
8. Flexor tendons of hand
   (i) Classical teaching — Burnell

Hand is divided into three zones

Proximal	Proximal to metacarpophalangeal joint	Primary repair
Mid-zone	Between metacarpophalangeal joint and proximal interphalangeal joint	Delayed repair since both tendons usually involved
Distal zone	Distal to proximal interphalangeal joint	Primary repair of flexor digitorum profunda tendon

   (recently hand surgeons have advocated primary repair for
   all three zones if both technically possible and the surgeon
   sufficiently experienced)
   (ii) Always repair flexor tendons on their volar surface since
        they receive their blood supply by vincula which are
        usually on the palmar surface
   (iii) Use non absorbable monofilament sutures
9. Postoperatively
   (i) Elevate the arm
   (ii) Encourage early exercise and active splintage to reduce
        adhesions

Index

Note. For the purposes of conciseness the most commonly described operative stages described in the text have been grouped in the index, when convenient, under the following subheadings: (a) 'indications'; (b) 'preoperative preparations' which includes preoperative management and pre-incision; (c) 'peroperative procedures' including incision, procedure and closure; (d) 'postoperative management'; (e) 'complications'.